Brain

Victor Serebriakoff

BRAIN

Davis-Poynter
LONDON

First published in 1975 by
Davis-Poynter Limited
20 Garrick Street London WC2E 9BJ

ISBN 0 7067 0105 4

Printed in Great Britain by
Bristol Typesetting Co. Ltd, Bristol

Contents

FOREWORD *page* 7

1 What is Life? 11

2 Intelligence 20

3 Cybernetics 42

4 Recognition, Classification, Generalization 51

5 The Motorium 75

6 Learning 80

7 Attention, Volition, Conation 89

8 Biomorphic Philosophy 104

9 Confirmation and Falsification 117

10 Implications 132

11 World Org 170

AFTERWORD Tinkering with the Works 175

BIBLIOGRAPHY 177

INDEX 179

Foreword

My principal reason for writing this book has been to rid myself of the burden of an idea. I have not exactly 'rushed into print'. The set of insights, if that is what they are, came to me quite suddenly and with an intensely strong (and frightening) *eureka* feeling in 1956. I wrote the first few sketchy and tentative papers on the subject in 1957 and 1958. A vastly condensed version of one of them was published in *The Scientist Speculates* which was edited by my friend Professor Jack Good. I have been fitting my reading, thinking and writing on the subject into an exceptionally busy life ever since. I know I have done only a fraction of the research and reading which is necessary to justify my intrusion as an outsider, into this field. But evidence accumulated, predictions which resulted from my hypothesis were fulfilled and I felt an increasingly strong feeling that I had a duty to communicate what I had come to for anything it might be worth. Perhaps there are *no* experts trained to pull together the scattering starting points in the very broad field I have chosen. I have written for the intelligent layman who remains the last association area of the brain of Mankind. I have not read enough to be able to claim that the model I propose is new and it must be for the expert in various disciplines to say whether it is true, or useful or at least seminal in that it indicates an approach or modality of thinking which has some novelty. At the worst it represents and possibly even presents for the first time a tenable way of looking at organization centres in their various contexts and at models of mental action, which fits sufficiently well to show that a physical explanation is at least possible. If it proves to be a foundation upon which a more elaborate and viable structure can be built it is surely the most that I, as an outsider, can hope to contribute. For my part I shall be glad to get it out of my system and I await its reception with equanimity. If it is not ignored I shall be pleased; if it is dignified by criticism from experts I shall be delighted and in the improbable event that it is taken seriously I shall be overwhelmed. What I do hope is to propose a model for mental activity for brain, in the cell, the animal and in society.

The model I propose is one that runs counter to many cherished modern ideas. So let us clear the ground. The purist academics I cannot hope to please. I am a generalist, if anything, and they are specialists. My model points politically to a conservative conclusion, which will be unpopular. Worse, it gives credence to the value of authority which leaves me without a friend or reader under twenty-five years old. But let the Conservatives be not too much comforted. I speak about the need for a dynamic meta-homeostatic stability of roles and the relationship between roles. I am not concerned with the incumbents of those roles. But I am concerned with the problems of the best allocation of those roles. (They should certainly not be allocated on the basis of social class.) From the point of view from which I argue, a role is a node, gate, locus or connective centre, in an information and instruction transducing system. A role is a relationship with communicational connections with a set of other roles. Certain roles, I believe I can show, must in any properly organized system have a greater informational and instructional 'weight' than others, and the incumbents should be chosen according to their ability to deal with the associated problems.

And while I deny too much comfort to the Conservatives, let not the Liberals, Progressives, Socialists and Communists write me off as a dyed-in-the-wool reactionary Conservative. My starting point was the same as yours. I was a Social Democrat, believing in a planned and ordered society. I do not believe in revolutionary change because it is uncomfortable and rarely necessary. But I now believe that we should look much more carefully at organizational structures and systems: at sets of role relationships before we tear them to pieces. They may have functions we do not understand. Even if humanity is a self organizing system, as it must be unless some God or Master Mind is running the show, it does not follow that we understand how it works, any more than the individual neuron in the brain understands how the whole brain works. Let us go carefully with our hammer of reform, and ask ourselves why an institution got there and survived before we rip it out and throw it away. To my Communist and Socialist readers I say: 'Persevere. There may be comfort for you yet in these pages.'

But if there should chance to be among my readers an anarchist who has not rejected the book because of its title, I have little comfort for you. No one likes to be confronted with contrary evidence. My advice to you is to get off this bus now: it is not for you unless you are stoic or masochistic enough to take on the mammoth task of trying to comprehend a directly contrary view. There is yet time: shut the page and re-read Malatesta, Proudhon and Kropotkin. You will find comfort there. I love anarchists and their talk, so I do not want to offend them. Go away, good friend, in peace, happy in the knowledge that large, complex, cooperative collectivities of humans can peacefully divide responsibility, allocate roles and perform exactly, the millions of complicated, highly specified acts which must be performed to keep us all alive, by matey works discussions 'on the bottom level'. Peace and order will emerge from the Natural Goodness of Man Uncorrupted by Institutions. You have given your credulity a mammoth task, further reading here is an additional burden you would be wise not to risk.

Now if I may resume my words to those who feel that organization, role allocation, the structured flow of information are, at worst, necessary evils and, at best, positively good things, in any society that hopes to survive and to serve its citizens with the best that may be available I say:

Most of you are living in a comfortable society where, by and large, adapting Hobbes, there are 'arts, letters, society and, which is best of all, little fear of the danger of violent death, and the life of men is communal, rich, pleasant, human and long'. Certainly we have not, in our big world, got this everywhere yet. But it is very nice, where we have it, *that* we have it. All the signs are that this pleasant state of affairs is not stable. All pointers some say, are at danger. Early in the next century, if the feedback signals do not work and some of the ecological props begin to buckle, we shall have the lot in on our heads. We shall not, in the opinion of this unhumble scribe, solve the associated problems by faith, prayer, gut-thinking, emotion, revolution, destructions or universal flux or—alas! I wish we could – by the operation of the Natural Goodness of Man. It will be solved, if it is to be solved, by the use of that object described by the title of this book, brain. Humanity must use its brains. We shall have to think our way *out* of a set of problems where through the talents of some people, amplified by a competitive consumerist industrial system, we have thought our way *in*. We must close the intelligence gap. The intelligence gap is the gap between the intelligence displayed by individual humans in their specific role in some human organization and that displayed by humanity as a whole which, at the moment, is zero. Humanity as a whole is slightly more intelligent than a culture of bacteria growing in its medium until it exhausts its food supply and poisons itself in its own excrements. But not much. The only hope is that although mankind has not changed direction at least we can hear the alarm bells ringing. I had a lot to do with the building up of an organization called MENSA, a world-wide society of people of all social and occupational classes who are of high tested intelligence. It has attracted much odium upon itself because it stands up to be counted in favour of intelligence in an over-egalitarian age which equates ability and privilege – a very false equation. I have travelled widely in MENSA and I find that, although we are unanimous on little else, (we are dogmatically undogmatic) there is fair consensus on two things. Firstly, Mensans are sure that there is an enormous and vastly important problem for humanity round that set of concepts with the names 'ecology', 'pollution' and 'over-population'.

The second problem, largely acknowledged by this small biassed sample of intelligent humanity, is that, in the advanced countries to some extent, and in the less advanced ones much more so, we have not solved the problem of finding, using, training, educating, morally motivating and utilizing the intelligence of those who, with undeserved luck in the genetic lottery, have been issued with more than their fair share of humanity's stock of problem-solving ability, intelligence. The intelligent should not and largely do not see themselves, I believe, as an élite of privilege but one of service. They should not seek but should actively reject privilege so that they may gain influence, because it is the need of humanity that they should.

Chapter 1 **What is Life?**

MAN IS QUITE CERTAINLY the most presumptuous creature within his own purview and I am a very presumptuous man. There is no greater act of presumption than that upon which I embark. For the scientist equipped only with a few kilograms of grey paste in his skull to expect to comprehend, whatever that means, and predict the infinite universe is bigheaded enough, but to try, with the same weak instrument to master the *relation* between the tiny brain and the vast universe is comically arrogant. For me, an unacademic, autodidact outsider, even to utter on this field, reveals, I humbly admit, a certain lack of humility: but there, humility is nothing to be *proud* of.

A necessary but not sufficient condition of getting better answers is to ask better questions. My subject matter is brain, sapience, sentience, intelligence. I look at that infinitesimal part of this infinite universe which feebly strives to classify and order experience and predict its own fate. My examination will be unscientific because large, crude and general, I shall be looking the wrong way through the telescope to see macrocosmically rather than microcosmically. I look at the brain as the centre of any organised system and I am concerned with problems of government, management, organisation and control. In the present deteriorating state of the great world civilisation in which we live, there are, I believe, the most important problems and this must be the inadequate excuse for my presumption.

The book is a start. I do not claim it to be a humble one because I am not, as I say, burdened with the humility which is incompatible with my task. My most extreme hope is that the ideas I throw out might be or lead to useful modalities of thinking which might help a little towards a reunification of some of the diverging paths of our sciences and philosophies.

The Question

My first questions are not new. 'What is life?' 'What is the difference between the animate and the inanimate parts of our universe?' 'What is mind?' 'How can it comprehend the universe and itself?' 'What is comprehension?' These are my starting points.

The epistemological nature of science

Science, said Eddington, is inexorably epistemological. It is to do, always and inevitably with the interface between the universe and the mind. The world, the mind and its contents – thought, memory, ideas, impressions, are inextricably mixed. Any perceptive process is the outcome of an interaction between something in the universe and the mind which perceives it. It cannot be purified of its epistemological nature. Our view of the universe and our understanding of brain and mind must inevitably be distorted by the fact that the very act of understanding is a mental event.

What is living?

Accepting the epistemological limitation let me propose an answer to this question. A first look at living things shows them to be active, growing changing, ever in flux. A second look shows the difference between the living and the non-living which seems too plain at first, becomes hazy and vague on close examination. There is a 'smooth slide up to life'. On the borderline are entities which are hard to classify as either living or non-living. The tobacco mosaic virus behaves like a living thing in contact with the living tobacco leaf but it exists also in a stable crystalline form which can return to the active form again.

But all human definition is plagued by vague borderlines so let us move into the central semantic regions within which it will be wise to confine ourselves. I hope to show later why the hazy borderlines between classes are inevitably so. A third look at life shows something strange that contradicts our first view of living things as less stable than inanimate things.

Entropy

In the unsentient, inanimate universe there is what Wiener called a one way arrow of time. One can tell a later moment in the universe from an earlier one because of the continuous loss of organization or increase in entropy. Sorted, arranged, patterned, entities tend to mix, become disarranged and lose pattern as time passes. Energy tends to become less available, and arrangements of matter which are highly improbable tend, in the course of time, to degenerate into a form which is more probable. The second law of thermodynamics establishes that entropy, or disorder, in any very large system will increase with time and as entropy increases, the 'probability' of the resulting state is higher. The universe started by being plain impossible, gradually became extremely improbable and, by becoming slightly less incredible every day, may soon be almost possible.

Both the 'big bang' and the 'continuous creation' theories were created to explain why the universe is still highly (and improbably) *sorted* (into galaxies, suns, planets) instead of, as we would expect it to be after the operation of the second law of thermodynamics for an infinite time, completely randomized and at a uniformally low energy level: in the state of the predicted 'heat death' in fact.

It is not only at the physico-chemical level of matter and energy that the increase in entropy is universal. Social life involves the manufacture and distribution artefacts, of highly sorted arrays of elaborate, highly specified, improbable forms and arrangements. The process of living converts these to rubbish and sewage in which they are broken down, mixed up and made unavailable. The increase of entropy, however, although it is one of the most certain truths we know, remains a statistical one in the sense that it is only true of large aggregations of matter. There is another very important qualification too, which I shall come to.

Negentropy

Negentropy is the term used to describe the processes in which, instead of being broken down and dispersed, order is built up. Living things, looked at in their environment, behave in complete obedience to the second law of thermodynamics at the atomic and molecular levels. But they achieve, at second order, locally, a resistance to the breakdown, dispersion and increased probability trends which are manifest at all levels in the rest of the universe. Living systems are platforms of second order stability of form built up in apparent defiance of the second law of thermodynamics, at least in a limited region. A living thing is an improbable ordered arrangement of matter organized so as to resist changes in its form which would normally be brought about by forces from its environment: changes arising from the increase in entropy which is ubiquitous elsewhere. Most of the activity of any living creature is devoted to resisting, avoiding, countering or adapting to changes within its boundaries which are threatened by its surroundings. All living systems, as Norbert Wiener and Ross Ashby observed, contain many homeostatic or stability seeking systems which keep them, the living things, extremely stable (within certain tolerances) with respect to many variables (ways of changing) over relatively long periods. I cannot find a word which holds the meaning of this second order form retaining tendency of living things and would propose *morphostasis* or if we are not afraid to mix roots (or if we are, *morphorentention*).

Morphostasis has a price, it is bought at the expense of a greater increase in first-order entropy. Living things consume energy (make it less available) and speed the trend towards chaos at the chemical level. At a second level the price of life is pollution, which exists at many levels; at the chemical level, toxins, waste products and low energy residues; at the morphological or second order level, metazoa produce mixed up food residues, excreta and at a third level social organizations as I have said, produce mixed up residues called rubbish.

Mainly, principally and essentially, living things seem to be 'set' to defy change. They *behave as if* they were 'designed' to resist or minimise changes in their form through time. I say 'form' because in all living things, the contents change while the form remains relatively stable. The morphostasis or stability of a living thing is the stability of a fountain, not the stability of a stone. There are other entities, for instance human organizations, which are morphostatic with which I shall deal later.

Death

Death, the termination of the process of living is not as we sometimes think of it, the resumption of stillness, it is the beginning of an irreversible run-away change, a defeat by entropy of negentropy, of the form retaining process, morphostasis. In *Cybernetics* Norbert Wiener said 'the stable state of a living organism is to be dead'. He was never more wrong, and if you doubt it I ask you to spend a month or two in the presence of a corpse and of a living 'control'.

Life is the bit of the universe that is 'going the other way'. It is climbing uphill towards less probable, more ordered arrangements of lower entropy against the universal statistical pressure of all matter and energy towards more probable states of higher entropy. Death is surrender to entropy, resumption of change. But the birth, senility, death *cycle* is evidently itself morphostatic.

Argument from analogy is said to be dangerous because all analogies break down somewhere. When I point out that social organizations of human beings are also morphostatic entities I am not simply showing an analogy; I am putting them as I am entitled to do, a valid, defined class of entities. It is legitimate to classify nature in any way we wish, providing the classifications can be used in an explicative or predictive way. We have no popular word for the class of morphostatic or morphorententive entities. The unpopular word 'org' has been proposed and I adopt it reluctantly despite its ugliness. The reader may prefer the neologisms 'morphoretentor' 'morphostat' and may read these for 'org' wherever I use it.

We could define an org as a member of that class of entities, including organisms and organizations which are 'organized' but I would prefer to say: 'that class of entities or systems which are organized so that they minimise irreversible changes in their form other than those changes which increase their power to minimise future changes'. Orgs are homeostatic, they (appear to) resist or avoid many forces in the universe around them which threaten the continuity through time of their form; they appear to act to avoid disarrangement of their parts, centres or communications flow. But they accept a certain special type of irreversible change and may often have special sub-organizations within them which generate irreversible changes which may be of this special type. The special type of changes which are acceptable are changes towards higher orders of stability. They are more than homeostatic (stability seeking); they are metahomeostatic (they seek better homeostatic systems). Into the class org I suggest we can usefully put all living things from viruses through protozoa (one-celled creatures) metazoa (many-celled creatures) organisms, flocks, herds, swarms, tribes, nations, organizations, firms, clubs, societies and even certain human artifacts such as cybernetic mechanisms.

I am going to try to defend the suggestion that the principal aspect of all orgs is a communication system. All systems of living things and assemblies of them which act cooperatively must have a communications system and we know of nothing which could be called a communications system which is unconnected with living things. I use the word communication in the sense valid in a context of communications theory.

The persistence of orgs

Living things which seem to be the most perishable things in the universe have, in fact, a more obsessive fixity of form than all but the most durable of inanimate physical arrangements. An observer from space who came here a million years ago and who returned today would find little that is inanimate unchanged in form; the mountains, the rivers, the stones all are mutable. But he would find the form of the leaf of a maple, of the bee, of the blade of grass had been, against all probability and within narrow limits exactly and faithfully preserved.

I am concerned with the methods and mechanisms by which orgs resist change and the communication system by which they receive signals from the universe and transduce them into form-retaining and change-resisting activity. Form is the relationship of parts. My identity, unlike the identity of the microphone in my hand does not consist in the physical, atoms and molecules present in me today. It consists in my form and structure. My microphone has the same atoms and molecules that it had ten years ago but most of those in my body have been renewed and replaced many times, yet I remain undeniable me to the sorrow and regret of the unfortunates who know me. Heracleitas said that everything flows, nothing abides. It was a good description of the inanimate universe where the all-pervasive law of entropy reigns. He was overwhelmingly right, but in one small region he was infinitesimally but untrivially wrong. A minute proportion of the universe abides.

Life abides.

Homeostasis

I have mentioned homeostasis: it is the name given to the principal property of systems which 'seek stability'. The word, is intended to apply to devices or systems which correct a variable; such as the thermostat in a water heater or the ball-cock in a lavatory cistern. There is a variable which has to be kept within a certain range or tolerance (permissible deviation). The essence of a homeostat is given in Fig. 1.

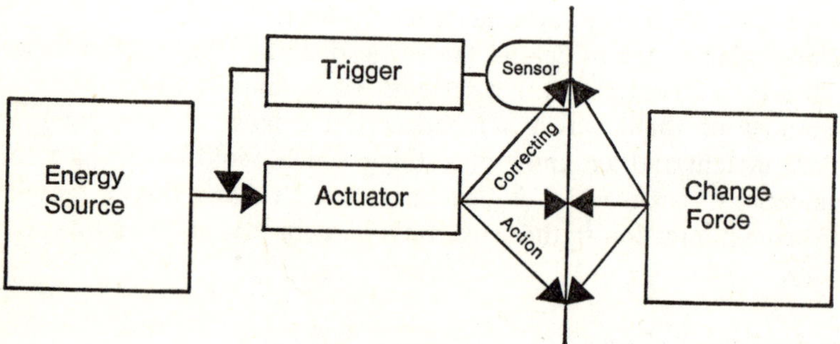

Fig. 1 Homeostat

Transposed to the biological context we should relabel the diagram thus:

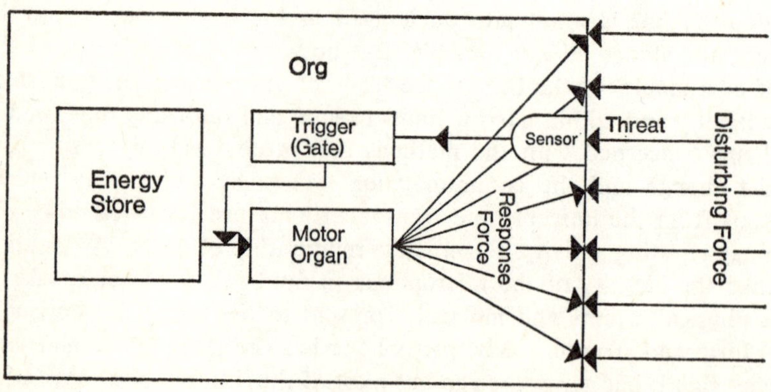

Fig. 2 Homeostat (biological)

There must be at least one instrument, which we may call a receptor, which is able to detect changes in the variables (water level, temperature). There must be a source of energy adequate to correct the variables and there must be a trigger by which the receptor releases the energy when the variables move outside set limits.

Triggers

The idea of a trigger or relay is essential. As the information always returns from the detector of the variable to the variable controller it is called feedback. The signal itself is a homologue of the change in the variable. A point that is often missed in descriptions of homeostasis is that the energy in the signal itself has to be smaller, usually very much smaller, than the energy required to correct the change in the variable. This is why there must be a trigger or relay. A small energy event releases a large energy one. No force can generate a signal large enough to encompass its own correction or reversal, the operation of the receptor itself must consume energy, so without trigger action or amplification the second law of thermodynamics would be disobeyed. A signal is a microhomologue event representing some larger event in the real world. For human beings, signals are the primary events in our world, the starting point of all knowledge, the input and food of the brain.

For instance the thermostat in a water heater is operated by a very small amount of energy, that required to change the shape of a bimetallic strip. The change in shape closes the circuit which allows a great deal of energy, relatively, to be released into warming the water. The energy required to make an animal's nerves fire is an infinitesimal fraction of the muscular energy that can be released as a result. A light ray of picowatt energy striking the retina of the eye of a buffalo from an approaching predator will set a whole herd of buffalo in motion.

I define a signal as an event selected by an org as a suitable microhomologue of some event which is, or might be, relevant to its morphostatic activity. A microhomologue event is one which is of low energy and thus detectable without damage, but which always or very frequently occurs at the same time as or before the more energetic event which is relevant.

Let us consider the problems of an org in its role as a morphostat. Its problem is that of sensing, detecting and classifying events in the universe which threaten, or might threaten the continuation of its present form or its power to generate similar forms in the future. It has to encode homologues of these events (turn them into information), store the information for future use so that it can be used in conjunction with immediate incoming information to counteract, avoid, transform or reverse the threatening events. From minute to minute the living org is looking at event after event presented to it and asking again and again the questions:

What is it?

What do I do about it?

Fig. 3 shows in a simplified way a notional animal adapted to counter four types of threat to its stability. It has, in effect, four minimal 'brains' and no coordination.

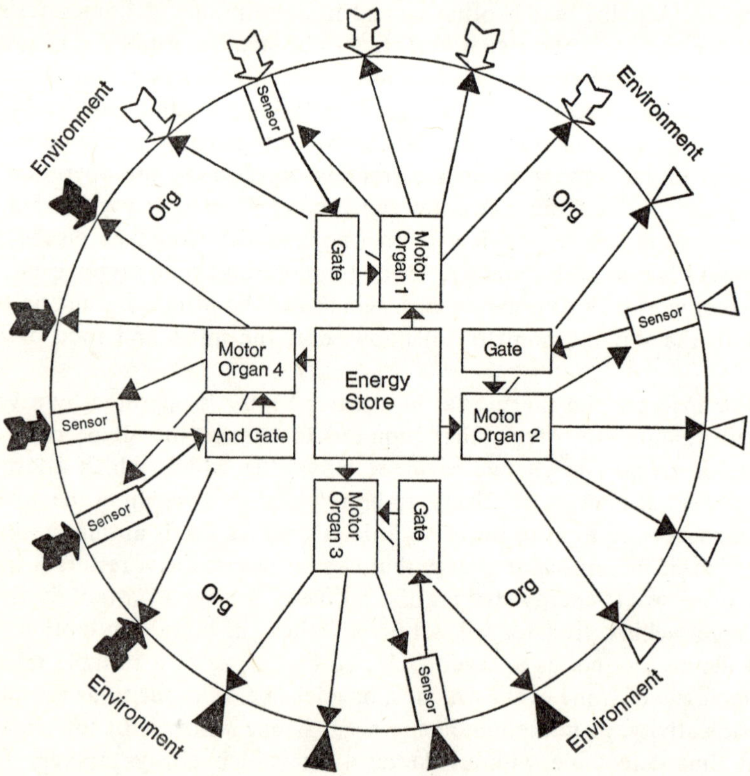

Fig. 3 An org or morphostat. Org threatened by four different disturbance forces has four motor organs triggered by gates receiving a signal from receptors (sensors). (Motor Organ 4 has two sensors with 'and' gate.)

Fig. 4 shows a more developed org. The threats to stability are not dealt with independently but in a coordinated way. This strategy makes possible the more efficient use of resources since priority can be given to more urgent threats. This is the primitive form of brain. Sensory information is received by it and energy released to the motor triggers after processing to a coordinated strategy. All except simple orgs have a combination of the two systems described by Figs. 3 and 4.

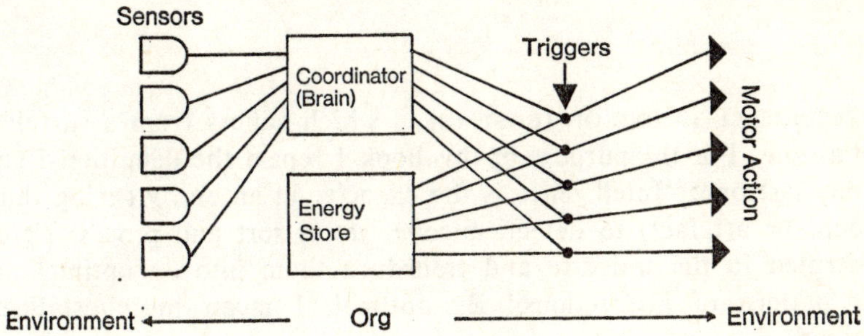

Fig. 4 Coordinated morphostasis

Chapter 2 Intelligence

INTELLIGENCE IS ONE OF THOSE IDEAS which suffers from a surfeit of definitions. For the purpose of this book I repeat the definition I gave in my last one: 'Intelligence is the capacity in an entity (living thing, group, or artefact) to detect, encode, store, sort and process signals generated in the universe and transduce them into an optimal output pattern of instructions.' By optimal, I mean morphostatically optimal.

The idea of intelligence is inseparable from cooperation. As soon as an aggregation of matter in a living cell begins to have separate functions, a system of communicating signals has emerged and intelligence is present. It can be seen at various levels. First-order intelligence is manifest in a cell. A chromosome is an information store with a line of genes or encoded instructions with trigger-like control of the development of the cell and its division.

Maxwell postulated a demon sitting between two containers of gas and opening a door which admitted only fast molecules into one chamber and only slow ones into the other, thus bringing about a disequilibrium of temperature in defiance of the second law of thermodynamics. Note: the demon acted on 'information' and made a 'decision'. A Maxwell demon in the genetic system of any living species uses information about the environment accumulated in past generations to trigger actions which enfold and entrap matter and energy into the recreation of a morphostat. Matter and energy is, as it were, tricked into sub-serving the continuance and stability of the cell and into rejecting influences which might destroy it.

The 'molecule' of life is a cell, the smallest living thing which can maintain an independent existence (viruses are even smaller but can only live within other cells). All cells contain many homeostatic mechanisms. From the point of view of information theory, the set of chromosomes is a vector or 'word' which may contain from ten to a hundred thousand 'bits' of information. (A bit is that amount of information contained in a binary [twofold] choice. One bit of information can reduce uncertainty by half. It can mentally split the universe in two.)

First-order intelligence in protozoa

Single cells, such as amœba, have a primitive sensory system. They receive information from their surroundings and respond to it in accordance with a built-in repertoire of behaviour patterns, these patterns of behaviour are, in some way, triggered or released by the appropriate environmental stimulus. Along the length of the set of chromosomes are a number of loci where coded instructions are stored. The instructions are complex and elaborate and they control the unfolding development of the cell.

In metazoa, different instruction-units or genes are activated at different stages of development, but since each cell in the successive divisions carries exactly the same set of instructions, instructions that are actually carried out must be therefore partly dependent on the information in the chromosome and partly dependent on the context. In one developmental context, a cell will develop into a liver cell; in another, into a bone cell. But something tells it which page of the book of instructions to read. It must act on information.

The Cell as an input-output information transducer

So the nucleus or 'brain' of the cell is capable of varying its output according to its input. It must have a sensory system in order to detect (select relevant cues from) its environment and so trigger appropriate instructions, just as the brain of a man or a dog produces different behaviour in different circumstances. The cell receives signals from its immediate environment; in the case of the embryo, from other cells around it.

The relation is deterministic at this stage. Any errors or deviations from the tree-like unfolding process results in an imperfect and probably non-viable result. There is little corresponding to adaption, or learning in embryonic development. The learning stage is in the fully-developed animal. Unsuitable patterns are eliminated at the somatic stage. The genes suggest, the soma tries out, and the environment accepts or rejects, variation.

Change-accepting mechanisms

Although there is no equivalent to learning in embryonic development, there is the equivalent of experimentation. Built into the reproductive system, of which the main task is that of recreating an established form; are a number of change-offering mechanisms which may appear to contradict my thesis that life is morphostatic.

There is a class of living forms of which the somatic form is haploid (haploid means having only one of each type of chromosome). This leads to very much more exact and reliable reproduction, which at first sight would be a better morphostatic system.

Yet most successful, *i.e.* existing, species, are diploid (have two sets of chromosomes). They also have a cross-over system which is a random, shuffling process by which uncertainty or indeterminism is fed into the otherwise deterministic process of cell development. The chromosomes in the cells of the parents could be compared to two long, sorted hands of cards. Each parent's own constitutions is determined from some of the cards in one hand and some in the other (and sometimes by a combination). Both parents contribute only one hand of cards to the two hands in the child but before they copy all cards and divide the pack (each become haploid) each parent shuffles blocks of cards from one to the other of his own pair of packs (crossover) so that two *mixed* hands are passed on. Thus though it is certain that each individual of the next generation resembles its parents in most ways, it is equally certain that it will be different from them in some ways. The final carrying out of the instructions results in each case in a unique individual. Cervantes might have been thinking of evolution when he said, 'Patience and shuffle the cards'.

Deliberate variation

The system is set up to feed variations, usually quite small ones, into the system in a random but deliberate way. The resulting animal will survive and reproduce according to how well the fully-developed body is adapted to the environment as a result of the shuffling.

Now let us consider the first-order intelligence displayed by a cell developing in the environment of other cells during the development of metazoa.

Those sets of instructions, those blocks of cards which produce, in spite of the change-accepting mechanisms, organisms well adapted for a particular environment will survive and be reproduced in surviving animals. Thus the species, if not the individual 'learns' or changes the set of its internal information stores so as to increase its ability to keep its form stable through time. In the diagram I show the development of a metazoan cell from the point of view of the flow of information. To aid comprehension we are entitled to draw the chromosomes as one continuous line of stored instructions. One configuration of information received at the periphery of the cell activates one particular set of instructions only. A different configuration (a different environment), would result in a different set of instructions being carried out at different loci on our line. We may draw a box as in Figures 5 and 6 putting the information-receiving surface of the cell, its sensory cortex,

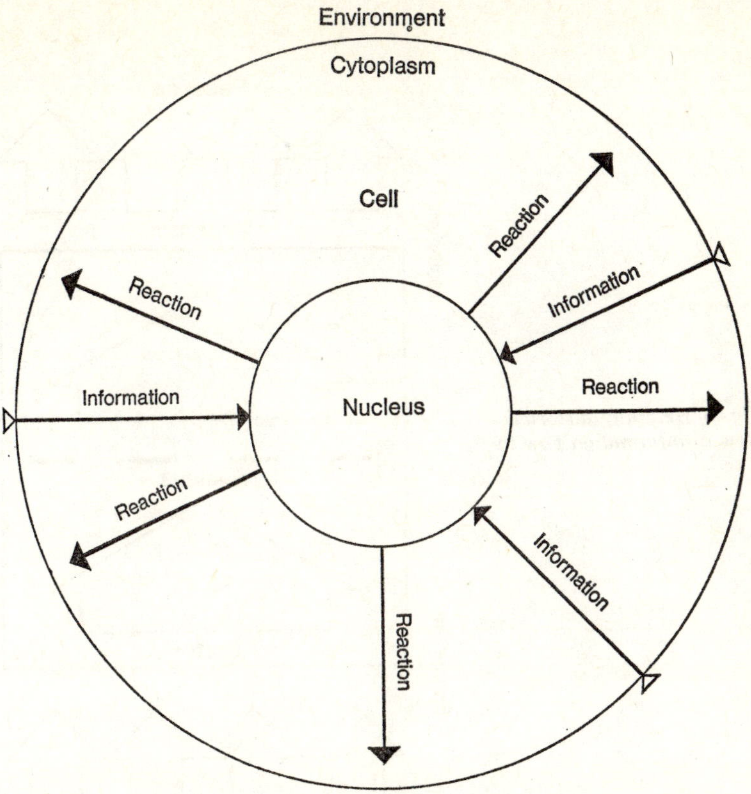

Fig. 5 Undistorted view of information flow in a cell. Cell behaves differently in different environmental circumstances and so must receive information and react to it.

at one side and calling it the sensorium. If we show the nucleus, with its conjoined set of chromosomes in the centre, letting the other face of the box represent the rest of the contents of the cell, the cytoplasm, which is acted on by the information in the chromosomes, then we can represent the difference between what happens in one cell and what happens in another under different exterior circumstances as shown in Fig. 7. A convergence of information must occur which activates the particular set of genes which must be triggered to convert the cell into the type and form that is required at that particular time and place in the evolutionary tree.

Each input configuration (chemical environment) produces a different effect by triggering different set of genes.

We may call the instruction-obeying part of the cell, the cytoplasm, the motorium. We shall hear more of this type of mental topological

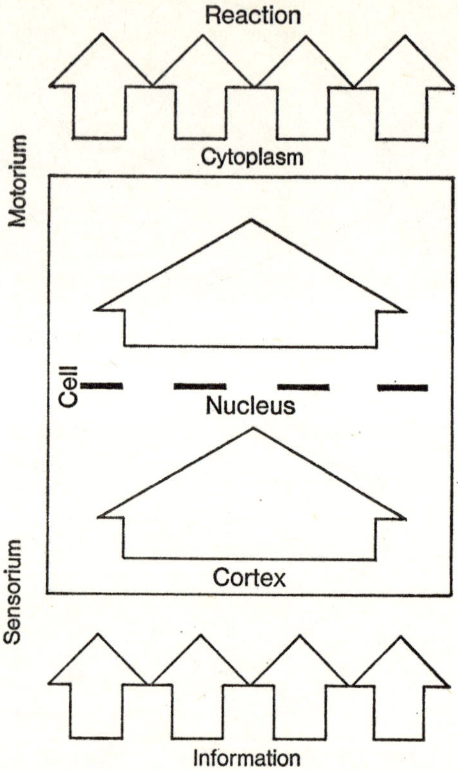

Fig. 6 Helpfully distorted view of information flow in a cell.

distortion later. Its justification is that it clarifies understanding. As information systems are concerned with connections and directions and not with spatial position it is allowable as a conceptual aid.

First-order or phylogenetic intelligence applies to the whole species whereas second-order or ontogenetic intelligence, which I shall deal with next, operates in the individual animal also. First order intelligence is a repertoire of discriminations and responses, passed on in the chromosomes; complete and unalterable at the beginning of each generation. It is only in the daughter cells that trial variations are made. The variations decide the differential survival rates of the various gene patterns, the behavioural outcome of the species as a whole.

The 'brain' of a sub-species consists of the whole set of its cell nucleii together with their mechanisms of sexual combination and their cross-over system. In ontogenetic or second-order intelligence, the crude method of survival or non-survival is sometimes replaced by a more

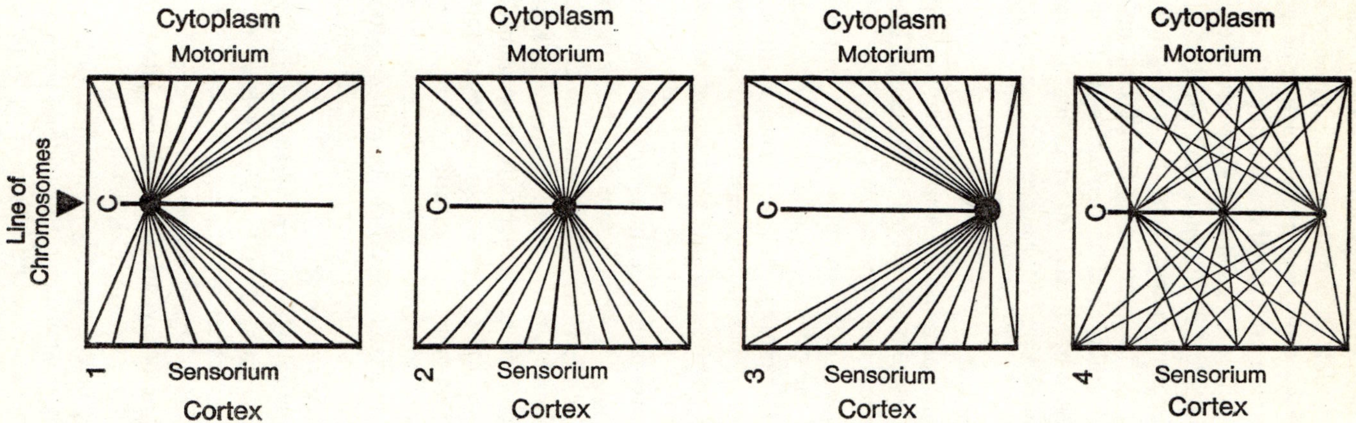

Fig. 7 The surface of the cell has been separated conceptually in respect to its two roles: 1) sensing environmental conditions, sensorium and 2) reacting to them, motorium. Information activates different genes (chromosome loci) according to the information from the sensorium.

delicate pleasure-pain, punishment-reward system which enables a single organism to accumulate information and experience appropriate to its specific corner of the ecological niche which is occupied by the species as a whole. There is a price for this advantage. The accumulated treasures of experience gained by each individual are lost when it dies.

In third-order or sociological intelligence, that which exists in groups and societies of animals, particularly men, this inter-generational loss has been circumvented by the communication of customs, traditions, science, knowledge and other cultural heredities. But anything that earns the name intelligence has a trial and error mechanism: a source of indeterminacy producing variety for acceptance or rejection.

Second-order intelligence

The more advanced type of metazoa usually have specialized cells which form a signalling system for passing information from one part of the organism to another, from one organ to another: nerves. They also have specialized organs, called receptors, for receiving information from the outside world, and others, called effectors, to pass instructions to organs and muscles. In metazoa, such as insects, where an extremely large number of cells act cooperatively, there is also a complex central system of nervous interconnections, this ganglion of interconnections, this brain, is the information exchange system, the central library, control centre which corresponds, for the animal, to the nucleus in the cell. Just as the individual cell, when it separates from the mother cell, has access to a repertoire of chemical responses stored in coded form in the nucleus, so the insect has a complete repertoire of elaborate behaviour patterns which is largely genetically programmed. Very precise behavioural sequences are triggered more or less automatically by a 'stimulus' that is a particular configuration of receptor inputs. A number of specific information input configurations neatly and directly trigger a corresponding repertoire of output behaviour patterns. Sometimes a single receptor may be the trigger, but usually the trigger input configuration involves many receptors.

Similarly the motor action which is triggered may involve only one output signal, but much more often the signals have to be sent in correct sequence to many parts, organs, muscles, to bring about the complex behaviour required. The insect perceives a certain 'whole situation' and the appropriate behaviour pattern is set into motion. However, the number of different patterns is small. The insect has avoidance behaviour, mating behaviour, egg-laying behaviour, feeding behaviour, each with its own particular set of triggers and its own highly specific configurations of actions at all points. If we draw what is happening from the point of view of information flow, we will have the same effect as we had when we drew the information flow for the protozoan cell. The whole of the sensorium, or any part, may participate in sending a configuration of signals to a trigger in the brain of the insect which releases appropriate behaviour instructions to effectors. This results in the divergence from the brain to all parts of the body of a stream of appropriately timed instruction signals for action. In order to conceptualize this let us suppose that there is a locus in the insect's brain which has to be triggered for each type of behaviour. We then draw these loci as in Fig. 8. and we shall find that the information con-

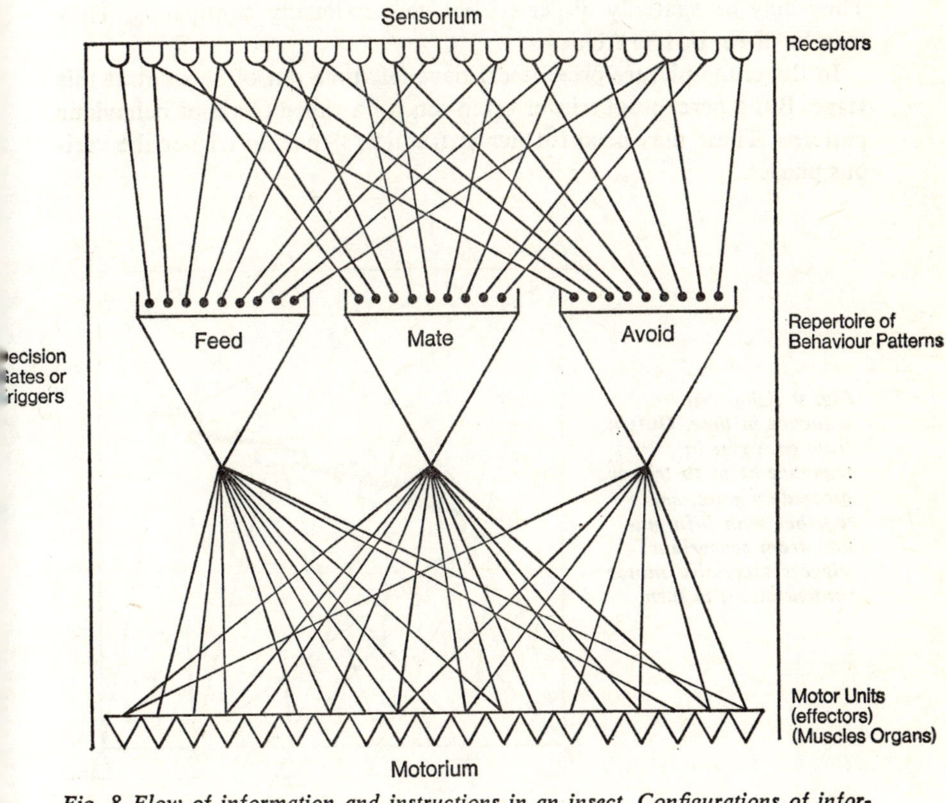

Fig. 8 Flow of information and instructions in an insect. Configurations of information from the whole sensorium trigger the appropriate motor configurations from a limited repertoire of behaviour patterns. There is little learning.

verges from many points on the sensorium on each of the loci and then diverges from all parts from the locus to many points on the motorium. In the diagram, for instance, information converges from the same set of receptors in different directions to one of three centres which may be where feeding, mating and avoidance behaviour is triggered. Once triggered, the information diverges towards the same set of organs and muscles. This is a deliberately oversimplified view. I am trying to show what must be the general path of the information. I am starting from the opposite direction to that of the zoologist and looking at the org teleologically; from the point of view of an inventor. Starting with a large number of receptors, finishing with a large number of effectors and having, from the same base of receptors, to generate a relatively limited number of effector configurations, the inventor would be forced at first to think of the convergence and divergence in the picture I have drawn. Whether the apical centres actually exist is for the entomologist to say. They may be spatially dispersed but connectionally contiguous. They may be direct or hierarchic.

In the crude picture presented I have left time out of account at this stage. But a perceptual trigger often sets off a timed chain of behaviour patterns. These may need further instruction signals to trigger the various phases.

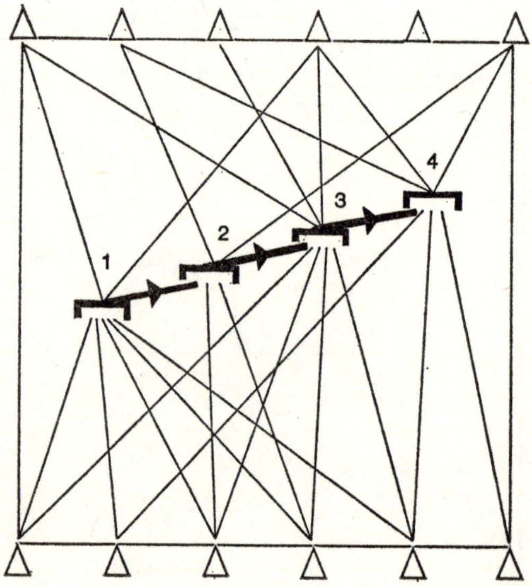

Fig. 9 Behaviour sequence in time. Output from each gate in sequence helps to trigger succeeding gates, and together with information from sensorium triggers successive motor configurations in turn.

Fig. 9 shows how this can be fitted into the picture. I have reduced the receptors to six, the effectors to six; a particular input configuration triggers the first centre, this activates the effectors and also the second centre. If this has now received the proper input configuration, it triggers second-stage behaviour and also a third centre which, if it has also received the necessary input, triggers its output. Note please that the triggers are what computer engineers call 'and' gates. They give an output only if they get all inputs (see p.62).

Vertebrae

Birds, reptiles, fishes and mammals have a further development of intelligence. Insects' intelligence is a great advance on, but similar, to first-order intelligence in that inbuilt behaviour is triggered relatively automatically by environmental information: there is a highly developed information-receiving system with a large number of complicated specialist receptor elements to receive it. Learning by individual experience certainly occurs but it is very limited, largely the selection of experimental behaviour patterns, occurs between generations.

In vertebrae, ontogenetic intelligence, or the ability to learn by experience in the individual animal, reaches a higher stage. Lotka (1922) said that the Biosphere (the living mass on the surface of the earth), is a kind of bottleneck in the stream of energy from the sun. All the energy reaching the earth is eventually dissipated but only after a delay (the warmth of the dead rocks absorbed in the day is radiated the next night). Life, Lotka said, interrupts and retains the energy, conducting it through the devious bypasses of the ecological food chains so as to delay more and more its eventual release into space.

This process, as I hope I have shown, involves the establishment of relatively long-term platforms of second-order negentropy, of unchange, in a universe of change. The direction of evolution is not only towards greater complexity but towards finding more elaborate bypasses and creating more stable and more complex forms from the energy flow. Huxley spoke of the 'barrel of apples'. The space in the barrel is filled by apples and the development of evolution involves filling the interstices with marbles and then those still left with buckshot, and so on. Every species finds and adapts itself to its own ecological niche. Species competing for precisely the same ecological niche cannot coexist for long, no matter how small the difference between them may be. It works like compound interest and it is a mathematical certainty that the one with the advantage will eventually eliminate its competitor, however small the advantage may be.

Following the barrel of apples model, if the adjustment to environment can occur only at each generation, it can only be to ecological niches which represent long-term, relatively stable environments. Day-to-day changes in environment cannot be taken advantage of. There is room, then, for orgs with a more flexible type of brain, a quick acting one, a system of connections between input configurations and output instructions which is capable of short term adjustment ontogenetically, within a single generation. There is an advantage for a type of org in which a built-in sensory event-classifying and behaviour-pattern-triggering mechanism (a long name for brain), can be modified to suit the smaller changes in the environment which take place within a single generation. Creatures with brains have the enormous advantage that they can move from one ecological niche to another as population pressure, climate and the general short-term ecological condition dictates.

All phylogenetically intelligent creatures are forced to be specialists. But ontogenetically intelligent creatures can be generalists provided they are prepared to pay the price. The price, as I have said, is that they have to start each new generation afresh with fewer built-in know-how patterns and less *built-in* power to classify significant events. They will need to build up stimulus-response systems anew in each animal. They will need a data bank, and a system for receiving, encoding and storing information for future reference. They have taken on the job of learning by experience in each generation so they will need it. What else will they need? They will need, ontogenetically, the parallel of the phylogenetic change-offering mechanisms. They will need an exploratory drive, a tendency towards experiment. They are designed to probe more minutely and on a shorter-term basis into the finer ecological niches left behind by the slow timing of the generation-gap learning system of the creatures equipped only with a phylogenetic intelligence. They will need something else. They will need a system to drive them towards morphostatic behaviour and towards the kind of behaviour, now no longer built in, which will cause the individual and the species to survive and they will need to know morphostatic 'good' 'viable' 'successful' behaviour from non-morphostatic behaviour which is the reverse of these. They will have to have a system of success measurement, a pleasure-pain system which tells them how successful they are in satisfying the now flexible, non-compulsory drives and appetites which have replaced the automatic (reflex) stimulus-response patterns. Impulses reaching the triggering centres will now no longer have an automatic connection with a repertoire of behaviour patterns. The complex patterns have to be *built up*, the experiences classified by trial and error. The direct connections have to be bypassed to new thinking organs. All activity can no longer be triggered from the mere presentation of a stimulus. Some internal 'drive', 'set' or 'appetite' must enter the picture to direct those aspects of behaviour which are to be ontogenetically modified.

The vertebrates, especially the mammals, have larger central nervous systems and rely less on built-in and highly specific behaviour patterns and more on generalized drive so that each animal has the power to adapt, there and then, to the niceties of its particular environment. It costs many lives when each animal has to accept the dangerous task of learning much of its behaviour afresh in each generation. But, in a world inhabited by competitor creatures with fixed behaviour patterns, the phylogenetic learner can adapt to their behaviour, while the fixed-pattern creatures cannot adapt to its behaviour. The advantage is to the animal which can predict without being predicted. The experimental, random, unpredictable behaviour which is necessary for learning has advantages also against a predator which needs to be able to predict the behaviour of the prey in order to catch it.

The reaction 'panic' has relevance here. An animal confronted with very great danger, goes into an unpredictable mode and appears to behave randomly. The species which has the 'panic' reaction might survive better because, in a tight corner, there is more chance that *some* of them would hit upon the, perhaps unlikely, but only viable behaviour.

Third-order intelligence

Third-order intelligence is organizational, sociological. It is to do with the exchange of information and instruction signals between groups of multicellular organisms, like men.

I want to explore the idea that there may be a unity underlying the three types of intelligence which has led to the concept 'org'. This is the concept necessary for the creation of a set of generalizations which may be equally valid for the organization system of the cell, for the many-celled organism and for entities consisting of many organisms such as flocks, swarms, herds, groups, tribes, societies, nations, commercial firms, clubs or any other distinguishable social units. This set of generalizations may also be found to have value with certain artefacts. Wiener pointed out the similarities between the modes of operation of control mechanisms (servo mechanisms, computers, predictors) and animal behaviour. Defects such as 'intention tremor' affect both. Since the publication, in 1948, Wiener's insights in *Cybernetics*, attempts have been made in many directions to set up 'inter-disciplinary disciplines' under the names Cybernetics, Information Theory, Operation Research, Behavioural Science and so on. I shall deal with them later.

The anthropomorphic model of society is very old and certainly existed in Roman times. Much of the phraseology of government is borrowed from the analogy between society, or the state, and the body of an animal. The centre of the state is called the capital (from the

Latin for 'head'). The very word organization comes from organ, meaning the parts of the body with separate functions. The relation is one of analogy and the analogy between a cooperatively-acting body of men and the cooperatively-acting organs of a body is obvious.

The set of ideas arising from this analogy proved to be useful and has been the basis of the development of the idea of central government. All analogies break down somewhere and this particular analogy, in a highly developed state, has proved to have many points of departure. In returning to it as I do here I want to do so in the light of much later knowledge. Since the expression analogy has become unrespectable, there is a tendency to talk in terms of 'models'. The human mind has no alternative. It has to encompass the unknown always in terms of the known. Good ideas thrown out of the door have a way of sneaking back through the window. What I am concerned with is whether the concept 'org' is a valid one. Are there a set of generalizations which cross the boundaries and remain true in morphostatic entities at the various levels I have described? If, as I suspect, there are concepts and relationships common to all living things, cells, organisms, organizations, and computers, control systems; then we may be able to fill in regions of ignorance in one field by reference to another. We may get the cross-fertilization of knowledge which leads to advance in it.

What all these systems have in common is that each has a number of information receiving centres sensitive to the environment. Each, as I shall show, has a source of energy and trigger-like mechanisms by which it is released into an array of 'effectors' through an efferent (outgoing) signalling system. There is always a central decision-making region, energy is released to the 'effectors' or behaving parts so that patterns of behaviour are generated which are related, at least in part, to the current or some past, stored, configuration of input signals. Advanced morphostats are also sensitive to the information in a storage system and to 'success' indicating signals. The behaviour of the complete system is morphostatic. It behaves teleologically; as though it had the 'purpose' of preserving its form through time with minimum change. My thesis is that where systems have as many features as these in common, there will be structures, systems and aspects which may throw light upon each other. Neurophysiology has uncovered much about the movement of information in the animal brain, but one cannot follow the complicated flow through such an enormously ramified system. Relatively, the brain remains a 'black box'. This is the cyberneticist admission that the complexity is too great for detailed description. But the much simpler orgs (from the point of view of information flow), firms, societies and organizations are open to examination. The flow of information is patent. It takes a form which I describe later. I offer the suggested pattern to the psychologist and the neurologist and the systems analyst for examination. But before I proceed with the development of this theme there is a difficulty that should be cleared from our path.

Meta-morphostasis

I am concerned, with the question of progress and evolution, with that class of change which orgs accept. The objection that has been offered on the rare occasions that I have exposed these ideas is that living systems do in fact change; by evolution. There is a built-in experimental system. Mutations and cross-over in the cell and exploratory drives in the animal appear to be change-seeking in nature. Both are vital to the continuation of a species but the existence of this mechanism is not evidently consistent with the hypothesis that living things are morphostats, change-avoiding entities.

But it is not random change which is *accepted.* Random change is offered for acceptance but those changes which are accepted are changes towards higher orders of stability. Paradoxically, those orgs survived best which preserve change-offering mechanism so that they can accept those which make them more efficient change-resisting entities. There is a semantic problem. If something changes, is it the same thing? In the case of biological development evidently there is a very important sense in which the evolving stages of an animal are the same thing. If we refuse to accept this thesis, then further ordered thought on the subject appears to be impossible. We speak of the evolution of 'the elephant' not of an infinite chain of transforms. We must accept the paradox of progress. Change resistance involves a special kind of change acceptance. There is, I suggest, a valid 'class', 'evolving elephant', about which we can make useful and predictive generalizations.

In human organizations, casual inspection reveals a high degree of innate conservatism. There is a strong tendency for organized human groups to continue on the same lines and in the same form. Incumbents change but roles remain. An organization may move from one place to another, but the flow of information within it continues in the same pattern.

However, like other orgs, the human social organization has a means of offering, for acceptance or rejection, experimental changes. In all orgs there is a constant friction and interplay between conservatism and reform. Between morphostasis and experiment with second-order changes in forms, which may result in improved ability to resist changes at first order.

It may be to some, especially in this age, a startling conclusion that what men and societies are seeking is stability. 'Growth' and 'progress', the ideas which obsess modern politicians, do not lead, as Professor Schon seems to imagine, towards a society in which all is change and flux. They are, by tacit implication at least, when looked at closely, a movement towards a more stable and predictable society.

We live in an age of accelerating change but it is not simply random change and it is not deteriorative change. Generally speaking, in a short-term view at least it is, or is intended to be, progressive change. We speak of 'reform', which should mean 'resume an orderly form after a disturbance'. Many politicians have forgotten that the principal task of the controlling centre of an organization, that of observing, classifying, comprehending, predicting and dealing with threats of change by mechanisms of adaption, avoidance or resistance, is one of extraordinary difficulty. It has to be performed against all probability and in spite of the relentless pressure of the whole universe in the other direction.

The whole sensory system of an org, whether animal or human group, has to be alert to threats of change. It must be designed and tuned to be triggered by the minutest sign, clue or pointer which may lead to the expectation of change. Orgs have no time to be aware of the normal somatic operations when these stable functions are not threatened. We are unconscious of the parts of our body which are carrying out their tasks normally; keeping variables under their control within acceptable tolerance. But if any organ, or the body as a whole, on any variable, begins to move outside tolerance; if the temperature, blood-sugar level, respiration rate, heart beat, blood salinity reach the alarm region near the borders of the acceptable deviation from normal; we know soon enough. Similarly, in our external perceptions the attention is magnetically drawn to aspects of our experience which are changing and moving. Especially is it drawn to those changing aspects which threaten, long-term or short-term, to cause unacceptable changes in our form. Or, to put it another way, to take one of the parameters of variation of our system through its danger point to death.

The basis of all knowledge, according to Hobbes, is sensation, and the causes of all sensations are the 'several motions of matter, by which it presseth diversely upon our organs'. He is so right, for nothing can be observed unless a change occurs somewhere. Sound waves are motion, light waves are motion, actual contact is motion, the movement of molecules of air on to taste or smell receptors is motion. Unchange is unobservable.

So while living things are morphostatic, stability-seeking, they remain so only because their perceptual system is excitably alert to movement, change and the threat of it.

Similarly, in organizations and societies, attention is paid to the unusual. If an outside entity wanted to understand the normal course of human life at any time on earth, it could be deduced by reading the newspapers of the time and place and drawing the conclusion that normal life is the opposite of what is depicted in them. 'No news is good news' because 'news' is a name for 'unusual events' and unusual events are much more likely to be bad than good for any morphostat. At second-order level only can news be good. It is good when it heralds the possibility of that relatively rare type of change, beneficial change, the change to more stable configurations. To this we give the name progress, or at another level, evolution.

When I first came to this conclusion I found myself, as a person whose views had always been socialist and 'progressive', very reluctant to accept them. It came as an unpleasant surprise to be forced to see that while the senseless inanimate universe is exciting, dynamic and mercurial, life (the bit I belong to), is essentially basically and permanently, boringly conservative. Many 'radicals', unable to stomach the conservatism which is equated with 'reaction', but beginning to see the impossibility of continuous and exponential change, have turned to support 'conservation', a euphemism which hides a distinction without a difference. More dreadful news for the radical is about that word 'reaction', which has been used as a ubiquitous hammer for all those who are not prepared to abandon each day the accumulated knowledge of the past in favour of the discovery of the moment. Reaction is the very natural and proper response of any morphostat to almost any change. It is another name for homeostasis.

At this point in world history it seems that, if we are to stand the remotest chance of counteracting and correcting the dangerously rapid and increasing rate of change in our world society, we must at least begin to understand that change itself is not a good, but usually a bad thing, and that progress or beneficial change is exceptional and becomes more so as development proceeds.

Geneticists flatly tell us 'all mutants are lethal' and that every mutation on the average causes one death. Their experience in genetics tells them this, because they find no cases of advantageous mutation even in the relatively simple organization of the unfortunate fruit-fly which seems to be the victim of most of their interfering match-making. While *all* mutants cannot be lethal, we can see that for relatively complex organisms, in stable environments advantageous changes are rare and improbable. The further committed an organism is in the complexity of its adjustment to its particular ecological niche the less tolerant it must be of radical changes. As complexity increases, changes which are acceptable and advantageous become smaller, less radical, more peripheral. The same applies to the acquisition of a skill. The rate of improvement reduces. There is a law of diminishing returns. An org, having got, as it were, the basic behavioural outcome or structure for a given environment or situation more or less correct, only trimming variations can be accepted. The organism has committed itself to a general form. Evolution has had plenty of time, ('Patience and shuffle the cards'.)

With continued development variations which are beneficial become increasingly more trivial until, looming at the end of the line for every species, in its own ecological niche, is the position when all but the most improbable advantageous changes have been tried and accepted. At that point, *if* the environment remains unchanged, then all change is bad. Only when competitive biological pressure or geological or ecological events change conditions can something which is both new and good happen. However, at the borders of every ecological niche is the no-man's-land between it and the next. At this point, where every species is trying to split into sub-species, the situation is different.

Humanity occupies a very special position. Man is a highly complex and specialized animal, but he has specialized in generalism and he exhibits to a high degree second- and third-order intelligence. He has moved into an ecological role in which he not only reacts to his environment but changes it. Man is something else again. Biologically he (and, for Women's Lib, she), is well advanced along the road of diminishing returns *as a solo animal.* But he has produced such a rich and strange variety of third-order orgs which live upon him as a substrate that there is no knowing which way he may go. These third order orgs, human societies and organizations, are at a much more primitive level of organization in themselves. As we can plainly see, human organizations can survive the wildest, the most radical and fundamental of changes, in form at least, for a short time. I am not speaking, of course, of people individually. Roles, not people, are the 'cells' of the systems and I speak of the systems themselves. They change radically but they are not very viable.

Particularly more recent developments in human organization are ephemeral. Worse, in the last six thousand years since settled agricultural life began, they have had, long-term, an unstable and ecologically unbalanced development. But more of this later. Geologically and biologically six kiloyear is too brief a time to talk about. I shall give my readers more information in a megayear or two.

What follows from the law of diminishing returns is that developmental and evolutionary departures of the most radical type can be expected more often to come from primitive forms which have survived without excessive specialization. New forms are much less likely to develop from complex, highly-developed and specialized ones. Progress of this kind is like the growth of a plant. The leading shoot has an unspecialized growing point: from it develops side shoots which successively lose their equipotentiality and settle down to some more adapted complex and precise role. A growing point remains unspecialized and spins off more committed branches and so on.

Let us look at the third-order orgs, societies and groups and combinations of men. These have developed, grown and built up their morphostatic systems on the substrate, as it were, of the mass of individual men and women. The existence of third-order orgs was made possible because one animal, Man, created a new kind of specialization. This mammal learned the improbable trick of sending complex trains of coded information from brain to brain. Man is the Gabby Animal – the one that learned to talk.

Certainly the most important difference between Man and the other advanced mammals is the complexity of his communications system. It is this power in human brains to stir homologous activity in other human brains which makes the complexity of human societies possible. Speaking and writing are very special extensions of mental activity by which relatively complex configurations of signals – information – can be passed from brain to brain directly. This is an improvement, even on intragenerational learning or second-order intelligence, learning by experience. This type of communication makes it possible to learn *without* experience, to learn by proxy, as it were. It is this kind of communication which makes an *organization* possible since it establishes the first prerequisite of an org, a communications system.

Speaking and writing is the sending from person to person of encoded experience, information, so that one man's sense impressions can trigger another man's action.

Conversely it is only within societies that the ability to talk has such a great advantage. This explains why the mammal, Man, has evolved to be so highly adapted for it. (The complaints of the Women's Libbers at the expression 'the mammal Man' are especially apt.) For the solitary animal the higher orders of intelligence exhibited by humans would be of little value. It is only because man lives and acts cooperatively, in relatively well-organized assemblies, that he needs high intelligence, and the higher orders of intelligence are of more use to the group than to the individuals within it. A Tarzan who really lived alone among wild animals completely without techniques communicated from other humans would need speed and muscles more than brains. The higher orders of human intelligence are useful only in a social context.

I once asked Hans Eysenck what was the biological advantage of neuroticism, why it had not been bred out. I forget his answer but it is tempting to think that it might be socially advantageous: to make people variable on a parameter of suggestibility, instruction-proneness, a built-in instead of fought-out pecking order system.

The strength and weakness of Man is that he is 'communication-prone'. He is highly sensitive to communication from his fellow men and, God knows, to his fellow women. The advantage is social, not individual. Suggestibility is the individual price paid for group support. I am indebted to Dr Jack Cohen for a story which illustrates this. In a certain primitive tribe there is a ritual by which the individual is 'bound' by having straws laid across his limbs. He is instructed that he cannot move and then he is beaten. If he survives the ordeal he is accepted as a suitable adult and allowed to marry. Unconsciously, the tribe is selecting for speech-proneness or suggestibility, because tribes whose members believe what they are told before the evidence of their senses, survive better in an ecological system of warring tribes than those whose members ignore stupid or incredible communications and refuse to cooperate in the personally dangerous but tribally advantageous (at that time) business of fighting to preserve living space. Societies whose young men react to gifts of white feathers by leaving the comfort of their homes for wet, dirty, untidy, uncomfortable and unsafe trenches have noticeably survived till this day. While, evidently, those from groups whose young men bow, accept the feathers and go laughing on their way have vanished in the dust of time. Maybe M. Hypnot comes in here. *Bonjour Monsieur. Pardon Monsieur. Au revoir Monsieur.*

But mankind is a special case. Risking errors of anthropocentrism we have to admit it. Man has reached a point beyond evolution. He has broken out of the confines of Huxley's barrel of apples. He is at present engaged in upsetting the apple barrel and is pelting the face of his Mother Earth with rotten apples, marbles and buckshot. The whole thing is getting into a mess and beginning to stink.

The total mass of the human race in kilograms is a trivial part of the biomass and an insignificant part of the total mass of the world. But it would take a lot of suggestion and a particularly suggestible man to deny that Men are the most important and influential part of the biosphere. The thing could be done but it would be tough going.

In the biosphere, the statistical weight is less important. As R. A.

Fisher pointed out, natural selection is a mechanism for generating improbability. The search for statistical laws in sociology and psychology is a lost cause, because living systems are a complexity of triggers, relays; Maxwell Demons which are out to defeat prediction. Orgs have control systems. The parts are not equiponderous. They have decision centres which act upon them and unpredictability is part of their stock-in-trade.

The evolution of Man the animal may be nearly complete, but the evolution of his organizations and assemblies has barely begun. He may cause such massive ecological disturbances as to release the full play of evolution up on him once again or he may learn how to generate new mutations by manipulation of his own genes, though he is a long way from this at the moment.

Apart from these possibilities, it seems likely that there is a ceiling to the development of individual human intelligence. This is illustrated by experiments in which rats were selected for ability to learn to run mazes. By taking the cleverest and stupidest rats from each generation and isolating and interbreeding the two populations, rats could be bred which were so far apart in ability that the cleverest of the stupid group was stupider than the stupidest of the clever group. But continuing to interbreed the clever group brought the experimenters to a ceiling which seemed impenetrable. They could increase the proportion of the population with the particularly good gene combination, but to make further advance the experimenters will have to sit out the long wait for a highly improbable new mutation combination. Or, as I say, start chromosome bashing and produce try-out monsters.

Senility

In the first part of the book I made the case that orgs are under attack from disordering forces of entropy in many ways. There are immediate, dangerous changes or long-term slow changes. The org has an extremely complicated odds-balancing problem in evolving the strategy to defer long term changes and counteract and avoid short-term ones. To find the best combination of safety and economy, there is obviously a relationship between the probability and frequency of a threatening force and the amount of structure an organism can afford to devote to its counteraction. An org must provide elaborate means to deal with dangers frequently met with, but the selective advantage to a species of systems to counteract infrequent, or improbable changes becomes progressively lower. Some of these forces are outside the organism, others are slow progressive changes within it. It inevitably follows from the above that despite Dr Alex Comfort, all orgs will exhibit senility. All will be susceptible to deteriorative changes that are too slow or infrequent for it to be advantageous to the species as a whole to bother to deal with them. Every adaptation carries a price and every time an org adapts or modifies to deal with one source of disorder, it is quite likely to disturb a hard-won adaptation to others. Only exceptionally will this be otherwise. Any engineer will tell you that optimum design involves a compromise in trying to achieve an optimum upon an array of objectives. The age at which senility appears in a species will be determined by the balance in the death rate from slow-acting changes and the death rate caused by whatever adaptations have to be made to avoid them. Since we are dealing with an extremely complex system it follows that there will be sources of change, deterioration, which are so slow or so improbable that the price of adaptation will be higher than the advantage of it.

Let me elaborate this. In the course of its evolution an animal must adapt according to some kind of cost/benefit system in order to deal with the many different threats to its stability which will confront it in the particular ecological niche it occupies. Clearly it will have to adapt its form and function primarily to deal with the most serious and most frequent events which tend to disturb its stability. Some of these disturbing pressures will be slow-acting ones such as the constant bombardment of the cells by radiation; others will be immediate dangers, as from predators. The decision as to which of the adaptive changes available are accepted by the species as a whole will depend on the balance of advantage and disadvantage from the change. It is unlikely that any change offered by mutation or cross-over will be advantageous in all respects. A thicker skin means a slower pace, an unobtrusive colour deceives both predator and potential mate. Inevitably, in an animal which is being cyclically renewed, the advantage of longevity in the individual is reduced.

Indeed senility may be positively advantageous to the species as a whole. It may preserve the form of the species by constant renewal which is only possible if the individual has built-in obsolescence to clear the ground of defective older individuals. Older individuals must be defective because of the law of entropy, any given event has a much greater probability of disturbing than of improving a complex entity. And time brings more events; more chance of disturbance, more chance of incorrigible disturbance. This seems susceptible to mathematical treatment.

A related conclusion is that excellence and risk are inseparable. In any set of orgs or even of artefacts made by orgs, like motor cars, there will be some individual examples which excel in this or that direction.

Those individuals which stand out above their fellows, on the balance of probability, are rarely those where the risks of failure have been kept low. It will be from among the designs where greater risks have been taken that more excellent performance will be found. And that, my dear reader, is why so many racing motor cars break down, why so many geniuses and would-be geniuses fall flat on their faces and why I have found courage to stick my neck out so far as to write this book. Serebriakoff's Law states that security and excellence are mutually exclusive.

Maxwell Demons

I am not advancing an animistic explanation here. The image seems to be a useful shorthand for the purely mechanistic operation of an optimization system based on selection from a highly amplified random input.

Chapter 3 Cybernetics

In 1913, an 18-year-old mathematical prodigy arrived at Cambridge, met Bertrand Russell and fell under his influence. His name was Norbert Wiener. Later, with his associate Rosenblueth and another group, he set off a scientific trend which turned out to be the first, faltering beginnings of biomorphic (defined later) thinking. It was he who revived Ampere's neologism 'cybernetics' and saw the possibility of a theory of information. Apart from being a mathematical prodigy he was an excellent engineer. The breakthrough for the budding would-be, interdisciplinary science, was the combination of mathematics, mathematical logic, engineering and physiology with which Wiener, together with Bigelow, solved the problems of prediction theory which made aircraft flight prediction possible. The design of automatic controls; the role of feedback in engineering design and in biology; and the statistical approach to information theory as well as techniques of measuring loss of information which are now commonplace, arose from his work. Wiener brought together a group of people who contributed largely in the development of computers. They were experts on control mechanisms, information theory and neurophysiology. Wiener, Caldwell, Bush, Bigelow, McCulloch, Pitts, Turing, Shannon, von Neumann; all were engaged in informal contacts, meetings and discussions which led to the hope that somewhere in the field of information theory lay the possibility of a unifying epistemological theory which would bring together the widely diverging exploratory roads of the rapidly proliferating sciences.

However, the initial promise of the exciting new insights of the period has not been fulfilled. The world has been deluged with a plethora of books, papers, lectures and information pollution on the subject of cybernetics under its various names and guises. The field has, unfortunately been invaded by many whose contribution seems to be that of complicating and bemusing. There seems to be a tacit agreement to judge the value of a contribution inversely in proportion to its comprehensibility.

Some practitioners of cybernetics who are listened to with attention seem to me to have much in common with the witch doctors whose aim was to impress rather than to enlighten. But those, like me, who believe that Wiener's insights were valuable and ought to be profitable, do not object to the army of cranks, outsiders (like me), obsessives and other intellectual oddities who are attracted to the field. New truths often look very odd at first glance and it is not given to us to know at first sight which of a large number of ideas are most helpful. We are prepared to turn over many stones to find a diamond.

We have a right, however, to object to the small army of so-called cyberneticists who deliberately use the interdisciplinary discipline to confuse and to exploit those they confuse. Because of them, cybernetics has no scientific respectability and even its devoted adherents tend to hide their contributions under another name. So many have jumped on to the cybernetic *charrette** that, at the moment, it lies in ruins at our feet. Some who were so impressed by its early achievements at the cybernetics conference in New York in 1946 have grown impatient with the obfuscation, the undisciplined ideas and exaggerated claims. We are now faced with the difficult struggle of rehabilitating it. Dr Rose has listed forty-three definitions for the term cybernetics and has come to the conclusion that the best definition is Wiener's original one 'the science of control in the animal and in the machine'. I would accept this definition if it could be extended thus 'in the animal, the machine and in society'. Ampere's definition was simply 'The science of government', and the first homeostat, on a steam engine was called a 'governor'.

The virtue of cybernetics was that it attempted a unified approach and used language which was equally appropriate in physiology and in communications engineering. One proposal, which I first heard at the Cybernetics Congress in Porto Alegre, Brazil, in 1972, was that the new interdisciplinary science should be called 'Bionics', the study of systems which are or behave like living systems; but I am suspicious of reform by nomenclature.

Professor Rose counted 1,150 different branches of science. They are divided from each other by the absence of adequate common language. The hope is that the interdisciplinary science of 'bionics' will help to bring them together by creating a common language of communications theory. The tragedy of this age is that the more we proliferate communication links, the less communication there is. Science has failed to solve the problem and the world is suffering from information pollution.

* *Charrette* is an 'in' joke. It was the little cart that collected students for the Sorbonne and so turned out to be a prototype Mensa; an interdisciplinary, cross-fertilizing intellectual group.

The story is told of the scientist who wanted information selected from the bulk that had been accumulated as a result of the lunar exploration programme.

'Do you realize we have a whole warehouse of records', he was told, 'and we don't know where to look for what you want.'

A cost benefit exercise revealed that it would be cheaper to send up a new satellite to get the information afresh than to recover information which did not happen to be classified appropriately.

The problem of science and the world society it serves is exactly the same problem that is faced by any organism. It is the problem of filtering and reducing a vast array of input information and directing it by summation and convergence to a set of centres where it can activate the political behaviour of humanity. The problem of information pollution is what I have tried to think about in this book.

The point at which information theory appears to have got stuck is the inability to deal with the semantic content of the communication chain. In its present state, information theory is a set of generalizations valid for mono-linear chains of signals being transduced at various interfaces. It is concerned with the mathematical description and form of the channels and not with the semantic content of the encoded message. I do not doubt that it will be the investigation of *multilinear* systems which will finally yield the insights we need, if we are to have a hope of using the information which is buried in the complexities of the world's communications system, as a basis for the policies and actions which will correct the state of instability and positive feedback (runaway change) of our present world society.

I have made the case that a distinguishing characteristic of every org is an information system. Conversely, it appears that wherever a communication system exists in a set of cooperating entities we are in the presence, at least in some degree, of a super-entity, a third-order org with its own higher order change-resisting systems.

The method proposed here is that the first step in creating a model, or mental homologue, of the exterior world in the human mind is that of choosing the set of isolates or classes which will be the elements of the mental system. Everything depends on the initial analysis. We are entitled to analyse the world in any way we like. The laws that will emerge will depend on the analysis we make. This was Eddington's point when he said that all knowledge was epistemological. Nature permits you to make your own analysis and she decides what laws will apply to it. You choose the laws when you choose the system of analysis; they were not *there.*

I propose to analyse sapience in the universe by looking at the movement, direction, type and intensity of the flow of information through the system, taking an unashamedly undeterministic, acausal and teleological view. I am looking for aspects in organizations and animals which will simplify the conceptualization of what is happening to information, how it flows, how it acquires 'meaning', gets sorted. I shall also think about discrimination and generalization in terms of hardware. From this point of view we have some difficulty in making a conceptual separation of the idea org, since the flow of information is ubiquituous and small orgs, form part of larger orgs.

The 'molecule' of the org called 'Society' is the org called a 'commercial firm' or 'association' and the 'molecule' of that is a role whose incumbent is another org, man. To look at each org separately, we have to tear it away from its two placentas of input and output connections. With our finite minds we cannot work without analysis so I shall perform the surgery by taking care to make our cuts at the places which give us the most explicative system. In this framework, we can say that any part of the system in which the information exchange is particularly rich and which is served at one interface with a large array of input connections and at the other interface by a large array of output connections is a conceptually separable org. In this sense the 'region' of information centres which are connectively or topologically contiguous may not necessarily be spatially so. An organization may be geographically dispersed without ceasing to be one. Remembering that in most orgs the number of information receiving points (receptors), and instruction transmitting points (effectors), is very large relative to the variety of decision-making possibilities at the centre, it may be thought odd to use our mental dissecting knife where it cuts through most lines, but I hope the development of my theme will justify this. It works when babies leave the womb. The complete separation is at the multilinear placenta.

Signals and Information

What is a signal? A signal is a micro-homologue event representing a macro-event or part of it which is, or may be, of relevance to the stability-seeking activity of an org. We may define 'information' as a configuration in time or space of signals which may move between different parts of an org. Wiener used the idea of Maxwell's 'demon' in connection with the idea 'orgs' which, as I have said, have to keep a large number of parts and aspects within small tolerance with respect to many variables over long periods of time.

Fisher said that life is a system for building up highly improbable arrangements. We can illustrate this by looking at any complex animal.

It will have a large number of parameters of variation, ways in which it is conceivable that it could change. For each of these parameters there will be a relatively small 'bandwidth' of tolerance which represents the range of viability. If we divide the bandwidth by the total range of variability it would define a 'probability' that that parameter would be, at a point in time, within viable tolerance. Each of these would be a relatively low probability. To find the probability that all parameters would be within tolerance we have to multiply out many fractional probabilities represented by each parameter of variation. The result is a very low probability indeed. But that picture is only valid for one moment in time. The probability for the next moment is equally low and the probability of the continuation of the org through time in a viable state is the product of the successive probabilities. So if we try to calculate the probability that all this complicated structure could come together by chance, and remain within the required tolerance for a few seconds, we must conclude that such an event is so improbable that we could confidently write it off as impossible. That such an arrangement (as a man for instance) can maintain itself with relatively little change for up to a hundred years, apart from the trigger-like qualities of the many Maxwell demons within him, would be not only impossible but impossible to conceive. By using small energy cues (signals) as triggers to control the release of large energy motor systems (muscles etc.), the problem is solved.

In the rest of this book I have to assume that the reader has conceded that the central problem, that of retaining stability, must be at least a major part of the activity of any living thing. The task is that of retaining with as little change as possible as much as possible of its form through time. I have deliberately laboured the point. If, at least for the purpose of exposition it is conceded, then the principal task of the information exchange, the black box, the brain, and of its properties, intelligence, sapience, are directed to this end, we can approach the problem of what sort of connectional system will serve. The essence of the problem of an org from moment to moment is this. It is receiving some gestalt or configuration of signals from outside itself at its receptors.

The universe is against it. The universe does not seem to 'like' the org's state of high organization. It is improbable and unnatural. Legislation has been enacted. The Second Law of Thermodynamics was passed and signed by God. The Universal Police Force, Entropy, has come to break up, disorder or make 'natural' all improbable arrangements. Defiant, disobedient morphostats are in revolt, climbing towards improbable order. The crime is punished; the sentence, death. But the revolt continues. The Second Law is flouted and defied. Life is the Universal Drop-Out refusing to join the proper natural trend towards disorganization, decay and breakdown. By a kind trickery, the very tendency for entropy to increase at the first-order molecular level, is used to decrease it temporarily and locally at the morphological second-order level. Temporary but ever-renewed and improved platforms of second-order stability or negentropy have grown up. The Earth's biosphere is seething with revolt, a whole region is full of more and more improbable arrangements, each becoming defiantly more complicated, organized and symbiotic.

Let us 'invent' an org. If the org is to delay breakdown, decay or death, for a time, it must have means of counteracting threatening influences and forces. Now, at the microcosmic level in systems involving a very large number of atoms and molecules, there is, in equiponderous systems (systems in which all the parts have equal effect), an enormous weight of probability thrusting insistently in the direction of increase of entropy. Quoting from Barton's textbook *Heat*, 'so we see that the second law of thermodynamics is true, and so very certainly true, merely because we are dealing with systems of very large numbers of individuals. It owes its validity solely to this fact, and that explains its wide range of applicability, for the law is a law which holds for any large number of individuals, whatever their nature. It is, in fact, a statistical law. It is definitely not true for a system consisting of a small number of individuals'.

By individuals Barton means individual molecules of gas.

What living systems do, as Ross Ashby pointed out, is to use variety to defeat variety, or as I would prefer to say, use and amplify indeterminacy to defeat statistical laws.

Barton was wrong when he said 'whatever their nature'. Living systems are possible because they have in fact access to Maxwell's demons which use small energy forces, 'information', to trigger large energy reaction in the direction of preserving the system. The org must have the services of a whole corps of Maxwell demons. An array of triggers for releasing energy into activity. Maxwell's demons (in the next chapter I shall try to guess at their nature), have to obtain and use information from the environment of the org. They have to decide among them what activity is appropriate and then they have to send instructions to trigger it. The energy directly at their disposal is very small. Microhomologue events have to be used to trigger much more energetic events. Maxwell's demons must have at their disposal an array of motor organs, each of which has access to an internal energy store but each of which can be triggered by the receipt of a signal at a much lower energy level than the force that it can release. The system is one of relays or energy amplifiers that can turn information, low energy coded representatives of events, to action or reaction.

An array of receptors, a central region of decision-making centres and an array of effectors, these are the first things we know we shall need in a brain. Not a very startling conclusion because all these things are physiologically visible in animals.

Now let us look at what our invented org can know about the universe. It has to examine it with instruments; and the output of instruments as Eddington has said is, meter readings, local intensities. Our receptor cells are instruments set to detect the intensity of some variable at some point in space time, some point, probably on the periphery of the information system. Eddington spoke of meter readings but one thing that computer technology has taught is that a meter reading, an infinitely variable signal, an analogue signal, which has to be transduced (in this case regenerated) many times at many communications interfaces or junctions, is liable to distortion. The preferred system has been a digital system: preferably a binary system where something either happens or does not happen. However badly distorted the unitary signalling event is, it may be tidied up and reconstituted at each stage in a many-linked system. So the inventor of an org would tend to opt for a binary system, a system in which information could be completely regenerated at each juncture along its path. What can finally be directed by the receptor instrument is the passing of a threshold, i.e. a change in a variable. The starting point of knowledge is point-intensities but all we can receive is news of changes in it.

All we can know is that some phenomenon has passed some limit, that a pointer has passed a point on a meter scale. From an input of signals giving news of these events, the org has to decide what is happening in the world and which particular configuration of its available motor organs has to be triggered into activity as a result.

I have proposed that for the purpose of this particular attempt at dissecting the universe we should tear the org loose from its connections at the afferent and at the efferent interfaces with the world outside it. (Afferent means inflowing and efferent, outflowing.) We could topologically distort an org (without disturbing its connections) into a sphere spotted all over with red and white dots, the white dots representing receptors and the red dots effectors. Imagine that each of the dots is connected, by a receptor or effector nerve, to a black box inside; the brain, another sphere; and we can cut it away until we have the black box in our hand with all its ingoing and outgoing connections red and white.

Now I want to ask the reader to perform a further topological distortion without changing the connections. First pat the sphere into a cube, then pull all the white afferent ingoing dots to one face and to the opposite face all the efferent, outgoing dots. We now have a black box in the form I want you to see it. There are some inconveniences. The proprioceptive receptors from muscle spindles and tendons have been dragged away from their neighbouring efferent motor nerves to the afferent face. But let me have my wicked way for a bit, in the hope that enlightenment may follow. Now we have all our 'threshold passing' news going in at one face moving towards our array of decision points, or triggers. After some complicated processing, they emerge at the opposite face to trigger specific configurations of motor organs, muscle fibres, or other reactions. Forget 'time', 'attention' and all the other problems for a bit. I have not.

What sort of quantities are involved?

For Man, the visual input from the retina calls for a hundred and thirty million white dots and for auditory and other receptors we can add about another million. Red dots are much fewer. We only have about ten million. You, my dear reader, have, from moment to moment, through your day to deal with 131 million messages shouting 'yes' or 'no' at you, and as a result you have to decide which million or so of ten million switches to throw. If I may be allowed, without being too effusive, to compliment you, I very much admire the skill with which you solve this problem. You may think that what you are doing is turning the next page of this wretched book, a simple enough action, which you can express in a few words and seconds. But the number of 'yes's' and 'no's' that had to be interpreted and the number of switches that had to be thrown seem to be out of proportion with this elementary task. And a poor cost/benefit exercise to boot.

Of course I have chosen a particularly difficult org as an example, but all orgs have a similar problem. Since they are limited by the difficulties of nervous communication to on-off signals they have to have a very large number of receptors to get adequate news of what is going on and they have to have a lot of effectors to give them a chance with the vastly complicated task of defying the great weight of statistical probability which is bearing down upon them.

Let us return to our black box which is already beginning to change colour a little since it has red and white dots on opposite faces. One thing is plain; that we have to find some way of reducing this vast array of information, of sorting out what is important and what is not. We shall also need some labour-saving system at the switch-throwing end. We have to arrange that the necessary groups of switches at the output face, we are going to call it the motorium, will be switched by one or at least a small set of switches further up.

At the sensorium, the input side, we must have summation and convergence. Towards the output, efferent, side as we get nearer the motorium, we must have divergence or cascade effect. This ties up very nicely with the introspectively apparent fact that we did not find it so complicated after all to turn the page over. The decision which was simple, somehow got elaborated into the complicated configuration of 'switch-on' signals which were necessary for the action.

So there we are, you dogged readers who are still with me. 'Point intensities', 'trigger action', 'sensorium', 'motorium', 'convergence', 'divergence', 'central decision', with these simple conceptual tools in your hands I ask you to come with me into the next chapter to continue our exploration of the most tangled maze in the universe.

Chapter 4 Recognition, Classification, Generalization

I HAVE EMPHASIZED the importance of triggers. Decision is the name we give to the pulling of the trigger. There is a situation indicated by incoming information, evidence indicates the desirability of a certain action. If the information is *sufficiently* indicative and *insufficiently* contra-indicative of the probable advisability of the action, a decision is made, a trigger pulled, a switch thrown, a command given and the connection between the sensory input and the motor output completed.

The simplest example of a decision in the picture as drawn so far was the trigger point at the threshold when some increase (or decrease) in the intensity of some phenomenon at a receptor causes it to 'fire' and pass stimulation to all its connections. 'The change in the variable I am watching', it declares is 'enough.' And the receptor makes the decision to pass information into the system. Now what is passing in at the sensorium of the org at any moment is a very great and complicated configuration of such decisions. The name for the process is perception.

Because of the vast number of receptors, the probability that any one input configuration of decisions would ever be identical to any other that preceded it or followed it in all time is vanishingly small. Each successive millisecond of sensory input is unique.

To deal with this difficult situation the org has to resort to the strategy of classification. The successive configurations, we call them events, have to be classified if the org has to have the ghost of a chance of dealing with them. Classification is the name we give to the process of reducing a number of decisions to one decision. We look at a particular configuration of input on the sensorium and ask the question does this configuration belong to this *class* or *set* of events or not. If the number, type, arrangement and many other features about the incoming configuration of 'yes' (or 'no') signals is within the tolerance or permissible deviation of a class (set, isolate, distinguishable entity, discriminant), the answer is 'yes', otherwise it is 'no'. If we have *enough* confirmatory evidence and not sufficient contra-indicative evidence the decision is made, the presence of a member of the class of discriminants is acknowledged and a signal passed on. As an example, the zebra on the veldt receives a number of signals from its ears, nose and eyes. *Exactly* this combination it has never received before, but it successfully classifies this set of inputs as 'lion' and flees.

Recognition

The initial, and by far the most difficult problem of the brain, is at the interface with the world.

The problem at the input interface, the sensorium, is the problem of recognition. Every perceivable total event and even every percept which is part of it is, at each presentation, as I have said, unique. Not only the whole perception of a moment, but every detail that contributes to it must be classified if it is to be dealt with by a finite brain.

Tolerance

Classes which have no tolerance or 'permissible deviation' have at the most one member and are most unlikely to have even one. The number of different configurations or combinations of input settings of an org with a sensorium of one hundred and thirty million receptors is $2^{130,000,000}$ two to the *power* 130 million (for the unmathematical reader; this is a biggish old number; indistinguishable from infinity). One of the parameters of a 'class' is the 'amount' of specification. This is the number of independent variables (parameters of variation), which

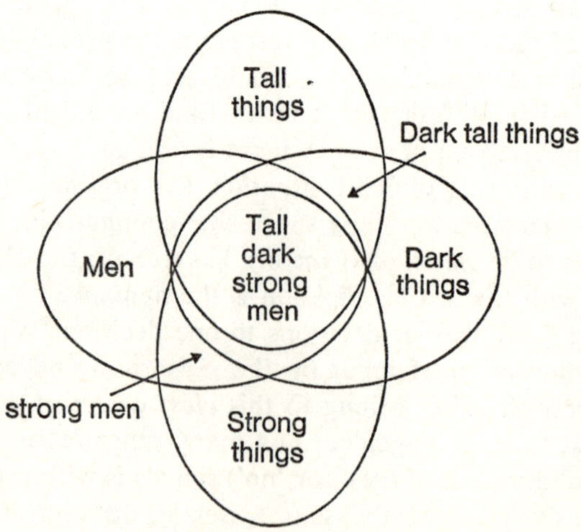

Fig. 10 Increasing specification

have to be within tolerance if the decision that a potential member belongs within the class, is to be made.

In the case of the configurations of signals at the motorium, each effector represents an independent variable with two or more possible states, 'fire' or 'not fire'.

The Euler diagram Fig. 10 shows how various classes of low specification, by overlapping, can create classes with higher specification. The class 'tall, dark, strong men' has more specification (and consequently less members) than the class 'men'.

Matching classes

A 'class' can be expressed in vectorial form. Every additional variable or parameter representing another dimension. The type of binary decisions which are received at the sensorium of a biological org could be represented by an array of noughts and ones thus:

000001
000010
000100
001000
010000
100000

This could be called 'diagonal line right end high'. To clarify, I shall drop back from two to one dimension. Let us suppose there is a doctor who has been asked whether a patient is or is not suffering from a particular disease. There are a number of symptoms *a, b, c -- n* which indicate the disease and he asks himself the question is *a* present or not, is *b* present or not, and so on. Sometimes the absence of something may be indicative of the disease, so he gets an answer like this

symptoms	a	b	c	d	e	f	g	h	i
observed profile	1	1	1	0	0	1	1	1	1

These are the decisions he has made about the patient. We shall call this line the Object Comparate, which we are going to compare with some model coming from the known symptoms of the disease. We may call this the Subject Comparate. Now suppose that the symptomology of the disease were exactly the same *i.e.*:

SUBJECT COMPARATE

a	b	c	d	e	f	g	h	i
1	1	1	0	0	1	1	1	1

in comparing one with another

	a	b	c	d	e	f	g	h	i	
	1	1	1	0	0	1	1	1	1	SUBJECT COMPARATE
	1	1	1	0	0	1	1	1	1	OBJECT COMPARATE
decision output	1	1	1	1	1	1	1	1	1	= 1 = yes.

The doctor has compared the two vectors and there is correspondence in each case. The answer is 'yes' in each case and the final decision is 'yes', the patient *is* suffering from the disease.

But very often disease may be present even if all the symptoms are not, so we may get a situation

	a	b	c	d	e	f	g	h	i	
SUBJECT COMPARATE	1	1	0	1	1	1	1	0	1	*i.e. typical symptoms*
OBJECT COMPARATE	1	0	1	1	0	1	1	0	1	patient's symptoms
	1	0	0	1	0	1	1	1	1	$= \frac{6}{9}$

So we get $\frac{6}{9}$ match, three disagreements. If the diagnostic tolerance is one-third, three out of nine, then the doctor will still say that the patient is suffering from the disease. For reasons that will emerge, I prefer to say that the 'sufficiency' is $\frac{6}{9} = 0.667$. Of course, the recognition of each individual symptom is itself a complicated business involving many smaller decisions.

We are looking for the primary oversimplification which will be capable of the necessary subsequent elaboration without breaking down. Where recognition occurs, there must be in some form or other a vector or array of observed decisions, there must be somewhere or somehow a vector or array of decisions indicating the expected or probable configuration of a member of the class and there must be, in some form, a set value for the permissible deviation beyond which the object to be discriminated will be classified as outside the class indicated by the subject comparate.

May I draw the attention of those with mathematical skills which transcend my own to the fact that these things are capable of mathematical treatment. The relation between the amount of specification (or the amount of information) in the subject and object comparate, the amount of matching, the amount of tolerance, or its converse, sufficiency, the number of members of a class and its possible variety and probability can be investigated. But to create and test mathematical models of recognition, we must first develop a connectional model.

In biological recognition systems of the more primitive type, the ability to recognize; the connectional networks required, appears to be built in. The new-hatched insect does not have to learn to recognize its relevant surroundings. It is born with the ability to do so.

Many birds and mammals have at least some built-in recognition abilities, but in mankind very little appears to be innate. The process of building up the necessary recognition mechanisms has to be repeated at each generation.

In the example given above, the linotype ensured that the information was presented for the matching process to take place conveniently. In the biological case, there is the apparently intractable problem of presentation. How is it arranged that the object comparate is presented properly for comparison with the subject comparate wherever it is? How are errors of scale, of alignment of register, and of resolution avoided? Let us ignore Pavlov, Skinner and the behaviourists for the moment and think about how recognition occurs in our own mind. Many objects, even complex ones are recognized at a glance. We can instantly name many, quite complicated, objects on the briefest inspection. But if we have difficulty in recognizing anything our attention is drawn from the whole to the parts. Like the doctor we look at the separate symptoms. If we cannot recognize a word we look at the letters. If we are doubting whether an object falls into the class, say 'cup' or the class 'mug' we start looking for the parts and aspects which contribute to these percepts. We commence a further analysis. Perhaps this clue tells us which way to go.

Going back to the sensorium with its 130 million decisions being made several times a second the central problem of classifying some fairly large part of the visual field, we have, surely, a process which must be convergent. Many decisions are being reduced to one decision at a number of stages. A tendency noticed by neurologists, called summation, is occurring.

If we count the number of cells in the optic nerve cross-section, we shall find that there are only a million, whereas there were 130 million receptors. Already, at the visual cortex (at the back of the brain), 130 decisions have been reduced to one decision by processes occurring in the retina and the mass of ganglia behind the retina. We know that the ganglionic cells behind the retinal receptors are indeed such collectors, condensers, or summators, or as Wiener put it, funnels.

Now, if we take this to be the first stage on a continuum, we get a picture of the converging direction of information which is anti-ramified or hierarchic. It is like a root system moving upwards. The number of connections joining at assembly points and from these, further connections joining up at assembly points deeper in the network. The structure is hierarchic in general form, but the direction of information is towards the apex or summit of each hierarchic level. Does this help with our problem? Moving up the hierarchic continuum, after the first

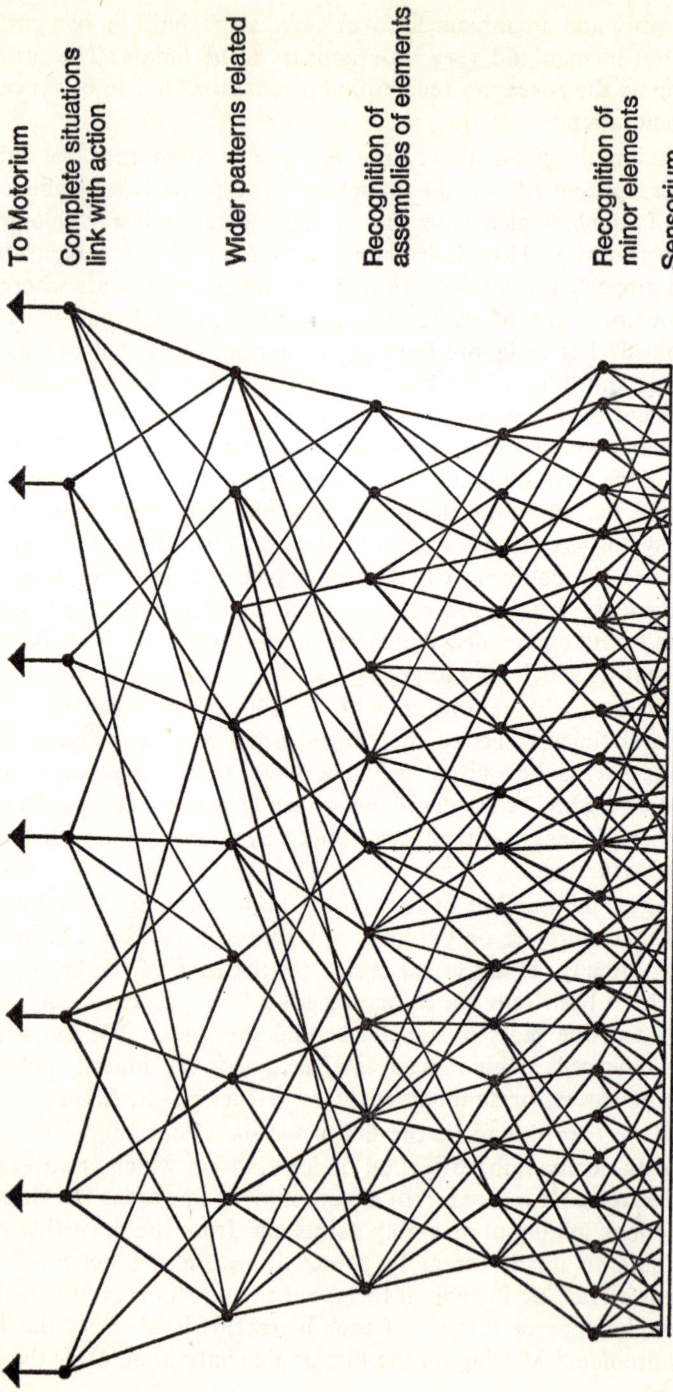

Fig. 11 A six-stratum polyhierarchic network

few steps we must come after a limited number of steps to a single centre. That does not help us much because many central decisions are made leading to many totalities of action.

As we saw in our primitive model of the behaviour pattern of an insect we shall need the organism to recognize a number of 'situations requiring action' and if our hierarchical system led to one centre we have solved nothing.

But does it have to lead to one centre? A friend, Professor Stanislav Andrejewski (now Andreski) in *Military Organization and Society* spoke of the structure of some human societies as being 'polyhierarchic'. The neologism defined a concept which seems to me to fit very well here. I would define a polyhierarchic network as one where a number of hierarchies, each with its own apex, spring from the same base. We have looked at the base, the sensorium and we see that the first step is convergence. Looking at the centre, we see many apices, each representing the assembly of the elements of a whole experience requiring action. Recognition, on this model, would be the process of discriminating, at the bottom level, parts, aspects, perceptual elements; at higher levels, assemblies until, at some apex, there are gathered evidence of the pressure of a complete 'event calling for action'. This apex must be the decision point from which an opposite hierarchical cascade of instructions must emanate. Fig. 11 shows a polyhierarchic network.

The model of recognition from this approach could be described as follows. At the first stage, at the sensorium, there is a division into functional areas; the retina, the tactile areas, the auditory areas and so on. Evidently the information from these converges because a combination of signals from any combination of them may produce a single perceptual result, the recognition of a single percept.

Taking the most difficult problem first, the visual cortex, it is suggested that the whole of its area may be such that a limited number of perceptual elements can be detected at *any point*. Edges, corners, terminations, straight lines, curves, motion, lines at various angles, spots, circles, no matter where they occur there is some post-cortical region which will say 'yes' to them and send on its message. I shall later discuss the kind of component which would be required for this purpose. Each kind of perceptual element is recognized wherever it occurs. There is for each element not a single locus but a whole set, a very large set, at this level, of cells or ganglia or cell assemblies, where members of the set of elements may regenerate excitation. The recognition of one of these perceptual elements is a yes or no decision. But there is tolerance. There has to be sufficient evidence that the perceptual element is present, not complete proof. If the element 'short diagonal line' is perceived, then not all the set of receptors on that line need to send 'yes' signals. It is enough if most of them do. At the second stage, assemblies of these primary elements have loci for their recognition. There are a large number of classes of assemblies which need to be recognized and each of them would have to be ubiquitously recognized. But since the assemblies require a wider span of the sensorium at the first strata, the total set of all the members of each class of assemblies is somewhat smaller.

Continuing the process, another set of loci at a further strata are programmed, by learning, (inductively) to recognize an even smaller set of 'assemblies of assemblies'.

Notice that the number of points in the network where a single percept of the lowest specification (a perceptual element) is recognized is very large indeed. As we ascend the strata the 'amount' of specification (of information) which is summated at each locus becomes greater and the set of loci required to represent every possible location of that object comparate becomes smaller. So at least we are moving in the right direction.

If we continue the process through enough stages, we shall reach a point where a very small number of loci are required to cover all the possible points where a complicated percept of high specification could possibly appear on the sensorium.

The optic part of the sensorium is highly mobile, is constantly moving, apparently trying out new positions and giving incoming configurations an opportunity to fit.

My thesis is that the recognition of a significant event (for any org) occurs in stages at an ascending series of strata in a polyhierarchic informational network. At the lowest level, simple 'perceptual elements' or 'features' are recognized as spatial patterns. Learning recognition involves increasing the specialization of a set of loci for specific semantic tasks. The set acquires 'meaning' by being programmed to respond to, and only to, the occurrence, within a tolerance, of the spatial pattern specific to it. Each locus is programmed to respond to the appearance of its specific 'perceptual element' in one specific field (which may, for instance, be a small area of a retina).

At a series of ending ascending strata, more and more highly specified assemblies of perceptual elements are 'recognized' by loci in higher strata which are programmed to respond only to appropriate assemblies. In this way a pattern is broken down and encoded. A perceptual element such as 'vertical line top termination' has a set of second stratum loci such that, with the appearance of the perceptual element in any field in the sensoriums, one and only one of these loci will regenerate excitation. The locus has acquired 'meaning'. Its excitation 'means' there is a specific perceptual element at this part of the perceptual field. A number of decisions about the grey level (local light intensity) at a number of loci have been refined into a single decision, yes or no.

When a certain perceptual element is present in the field or sensorium, there will be at some point on the first stratum a cascade of signals indicating the presence of all the perceptual elements associated with the percept. At higher strata assemblies of these, and at higher strata still, assemblies of these will cause regeneration of excitation at specific loci. In this sense, pattern is transduced and encoded as locus at an ascending series of strata. The flow of information is, in sum, both convergent and divergent and this is not a contradiction. For any one percept the elements converge to, at *each strata*, a diminishing number of loci until they finally reach the locus or small set of loci which represent the whole percept. But since there may be a very great variety of percepts to be recognized we have the situation as we ascend the strata that there are less loci representing a given percept but a greater number of loci representing different percepts. A relatively small number of perceptual elements will serve to help in the recognition process of a very large number of complete percepts and situations. Thus centrally we might expect to find that complete assemblies of percepts, events or situations might have only one locus where they can all be assembled and recognized. Simple percepts, 'spoon', 'chair', 'pencil' might require many loci but the 'semantic abstraction' of each might have only one. The many possible specific appearances of members of the classes described by these words, are all connected 'or-wise' to the final hearing, speaking centre common to all members of the particular class. This is the semantic or concept centre of the class. I do not suppose that spatial physical connections would have the form described they may be devious in the extreme and the set of loci representing any percept may be very widely dispersed, especially at the higher strata, but the connectional properties might still be of the type described. We should notice, and this is very important, that there is no limit to the number of apices to a polyhierarchic network. Each primary sensorium receptor can be connected to a large number of second stratum centres and a large elaboration of apices.

A three-dimensional representation of a simple polyhierarchic structure from a sensorium is shown in Fig. 12.

A successful model of biological visual recognition must explain the fact that percepts are recognized regardless of alignment register scale and intensity or grey level. In a primitive model of a recognition system there must be an object comparate and a subject comparate.

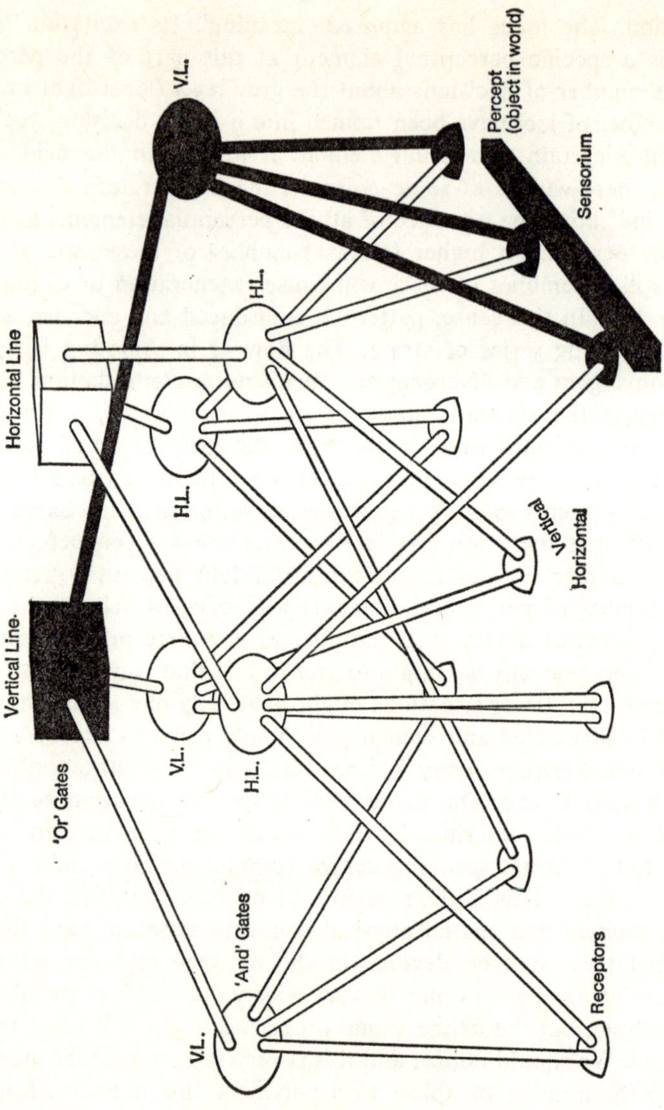

Fig. 12 A three-dimensional polyhierarchic network with 'and' gates (black 'VL eggs') for every occurrence of vertical line on receptors (white domes) and every occurrence of horizontal line ('HL eggs'). 'Or' gate (black cube) gives output for any case of vertical line and white cube similarly regenerates horizontal line.

The problem which I describe as that of 'register' is that of ensuring that the two match each other at every point and are not 'out of phase' as it were. Alignment problems concern the difficulty of ensuring that the subject and object comparate are not, one relative to the other, rotated.

If the subject and object comparates are not of the same scale there can be no recognition; a small x will not fit a large X. These problems are easily overcome by the polyhierarchic pattern for recognition. The problem of fitting the object comparate to the subject comparate is solved if the individual parts of the object comparate can be successfully recognized at any point on the sensorium. Similarly, if every combination of the necessary elements for a percept has its own recognition centre then problems of scale are overcome also since every assembly of the correct elements, whether widely dispersed or not, should have a locus or gate specialized to the task of accepting it. Alignment, or rotation problems are much more difficult and one notes that, for instance, reading upside down requires separate training. This leads on to one of the most difficult problems.

Any model of perception which is to be taken seriously has to deal with tolerance. I have to show how a polyhierarchic model of perception explains the enormous tolerance of biological recognition. This is my next task and to do it we need to proceed a little further with our task of inventing an org.

Deterministic computers

The general pattern of modern computers is completely deterministic. If we had a row of computers of the same make and we fed in the same programme and the same data we should expect to get exactly the same printout from each. A computer belongs to a logical determinist world and knows nothing of uncertainty. But let us look at some of the components of a computer, because they may be useful in helping us with the design of the information transducing system or brain of our org. The computer device for reducing two decisions to one decision is an 'and' gate. It is a gate such that it gives an output if, and only if, it receives two inputs. If both its afferent connections say yes, it says 'yes' and pass on the message. An 'or' gate is one where, if *either* of its inputs says yes, the gate says 'yes' itself (there are also 'nand' and 'nor' gates which work oppositely). 'And' and 'Or' gates are shown in Fig. 13.

By rigging up a number of 'and' gates, we can easily make a multiple-input 'and' gate where all of any number of input connections must receive an input if there is to be an output. Modifying this concept a little we may speak of a 'sufficiency' gate – an 'and' gate with tolerance which will say 'yes' if enough of its afferent connections receive an input. These are used, I find, in pattern recognition under the names 'voting' gates or 'threshold' gates. See Fig. 14.

In the small square I show the 'sufficiency' of the gate, the number, or proportion of inputs which are required to create an output. It is an

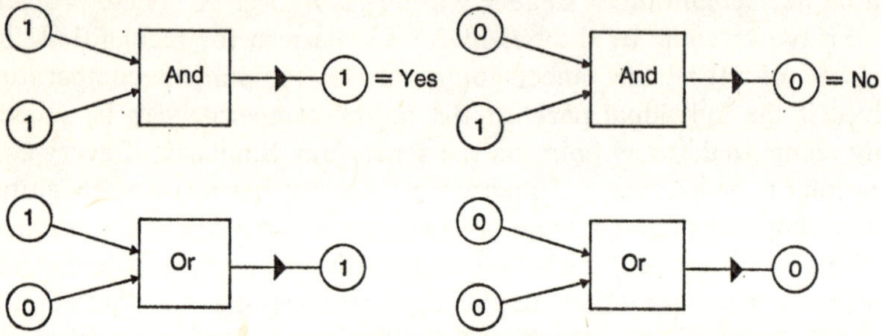

Fig. 13 Gates

evidence gate. If it gets 'enough' evidence, it makes a positive decision and sends it on. The doctor checking symptoms is acting like such a gate. We shall need such a gate to detect a perceptual element if we are to do so with some tolerance.

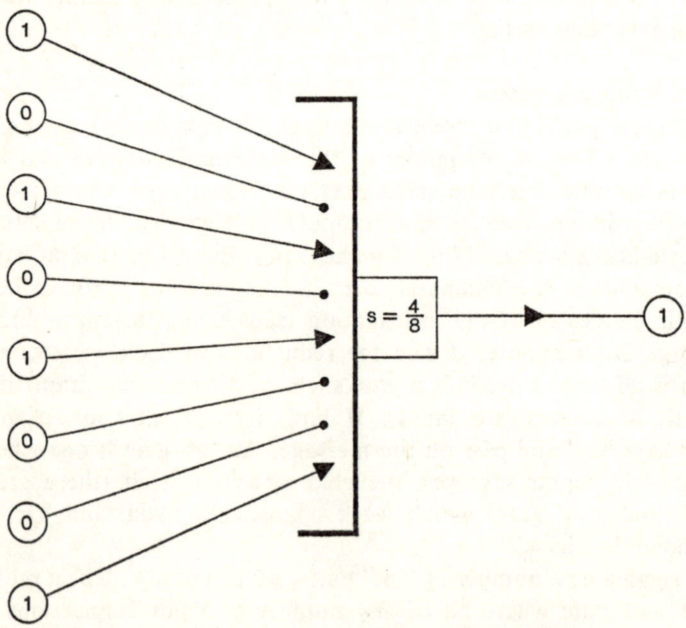

Fig. 14 Sufficiency gate (voting or threshold gate)

By introducing the idea of tolerance to the 'and' gate we have smudged the borderline between the 'and' gate and the 'or' gate. If we gradually decrease the sufficiency (increase the tolerance) of an 'and' gate with ten connections demanding ten, then nine, then eight, then seven, inputs to create an output, we shall soon reach the position when we only require one, and our 'and' gate has been transformed into an 'or' gate.

So gates can become more 'andish' or more 'orish' and this, we shall see, will be very helpful in explaining things about learning and tolerance and recognition. Once the initial work of abstracting the significant evidence of experience has been accomplished at the lower strata where gates would be rather 'andish' and have high sufficiency, we could, if we liked, allow the gates at higher strata to become more 'orish' so that many different presentations of members of a class of percepts could still excite a particular locus or set of loci. We shall need a component something like an 'or' gate when we come to consider the process of generalization. Up till now we have spoken only of receptors which send a 'yes' signal, or rather we have spoken of the transmission of a signal and compared it with a state of non-transmission. But signals can be of two kinds. They can be indicative or contra-indicative, excitatory or inhibitive, they can say yes or they can say no. The final version of the gate we shall need, which can learn to form a polyhierarchic recognition network, is a sufficiency gate where the input signals can have three states, yes, no or neutral (the signal has excitatory, inhibitory or no effect on gate). We then have a gate where, if the number of positive inputs it receives exceeds the number of negative inputs it receives by a 'sufficient' margin, it will regenerate a signal and send it to all its efferent connections. To some it may send positive excitatory signals, to others it may send negative, inhibitive ones. And along other connections it may pass no message. To show how an 'and' gate could be used in a connection system to recognize the appearance of perceptual elements at any point on a sensorium the reader is asked to look at Fig. 15. At the base of the diagram is a sensorium of pairs of receptors. Four 'and' gates are arranged to recognize a line wherever it appears and another four 'and' gates will recognize a dot anywhere. The receptors are in pairs and one can detect the presence of the line and send a signal if they do; others are 'off' receptors and send a signal if they see 'non-line' or a space. The receptors are grouped in pairs to simplify understanding. Perception of the signal 'dot' '010' must excite one of the 'dot' gates because every possible arrangement of '010' leads to an 'and' gate. Similarly the three positions where 'line' '0110' can be placed lead to another set of 'and'

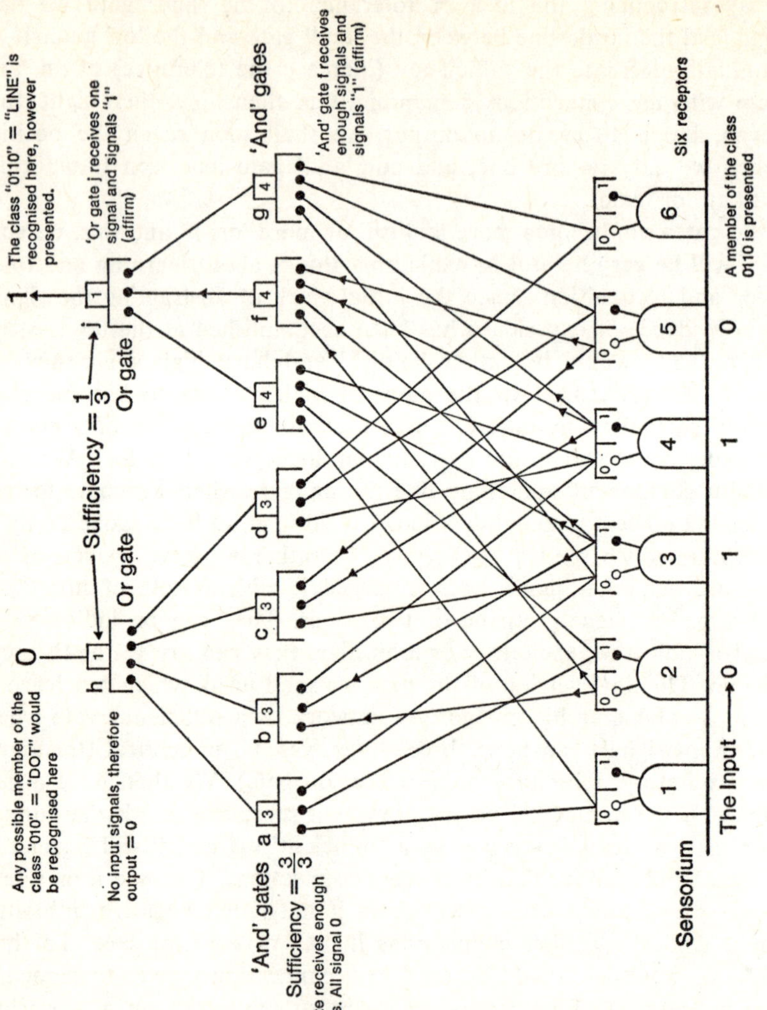

Fig. 15 Generalization – a recognition network for the classes '010' and '0110'. This network will recognize any member of these classes anywhere on the sensorium.

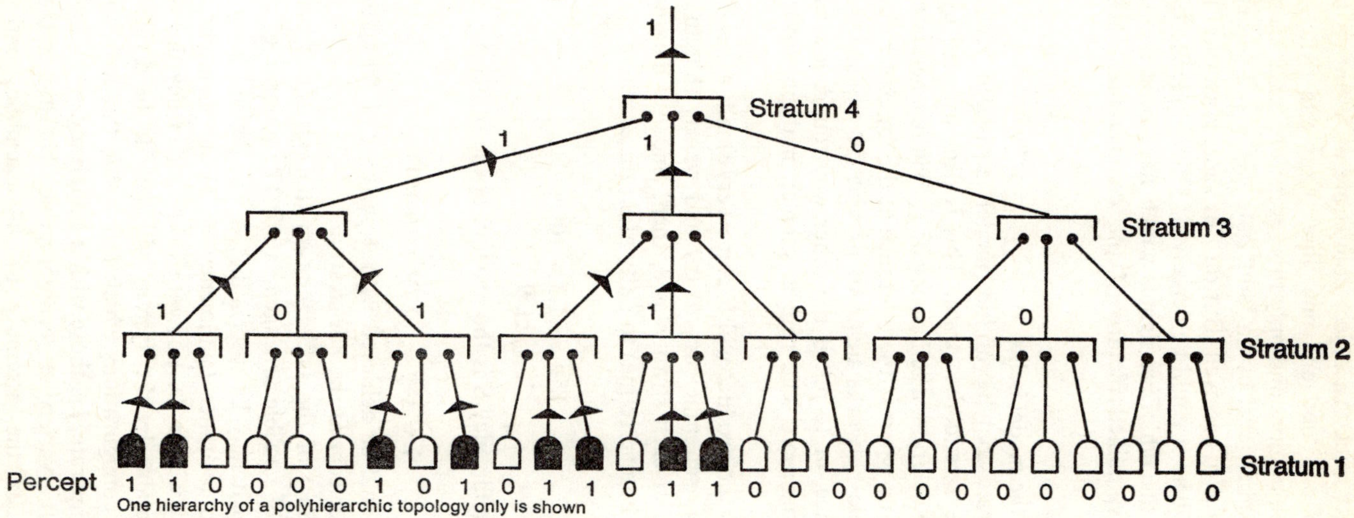

Fig. 16 How recognition can have wide tolerance. Sufficiency diminishes at higher strata. Sufficiency at Stratum 1 (sensorium) is ^{3}, *but at Stratum 4 (apex) it is* $(\frac{2}{3})^3 = \frac{8}{27}$. *The rule is: The sufficiency at a stratum with respect to a stratum below it is the product of the sufficiencies at all the interposed strata.*

gates at the lowest level. An object comparate or 'event' is presented which consists of one 'dot' and one 'line'. Only one gate receives a signal on all incoming lines and only this regenerates excitation. But all are joined at a higher level by an 'and' gate where the percept 'space dot space line space' is received. But on this short sensorium there are only 3 positions where it could be perceived. This simple model is without tolerance or the inhibitive signals which have been mentioned. It provides a first simplified picture of the connectional network envisaged.

Tolerance How the model helps

In the many-strata polyhierarchic model envisaged, tolerance is cumulative as we ascend the strata. This is demonstrated by Fig. 16 As is shown in the diagram, a sufficiency of $\frac{8}{29}$ will regenerate excitation at the third stratum, whereas the tolerance at the lowest stratum is 2/3. The polyhierarchic networks helps to provide an explanation of the very wide tolerance, or to put it the other way round, low sufficiency of biological recognition. The rule is simple: multiply sufficiency at the various strata.

Being fractions the product will become very small, a few strata up. For instance if we set sufficiency at 0.7 and we say that the average number of inputs at each stratum is 8, then, since we have to reduce 1.3×10^8 (for the human retina) to unity at S_m stages where S_m = number of strata

$$8^{S_m} = 1.3 \times 10^8$$
$$\therefore s_m \simeq 9$$

Now since total sufficiency S is the product of the sufficiency s at each stratum we get

$$S = s^{S_m} = (0.7)^9 = 0.0403$$

i.e. recognition could be achieved with 4 per cent of the pattern or a tolerance of 96 per cent at the 8th stratum.

What is the effect of the sufficiency on the amount of perceivable variety (number of possible arrangements)? The number of classes of configuration which may be discriminated will depend upon the sufficiency. With no tolerance (sufficiency = 1) and n inputs, the discriminable variety will be 2^n. But with lower sufficiency the variety of classes discriminatable by the system will have to be divided by the variety of object configurations which fall within the class boundaries of the subject comparate, *i.e.* those within sufficiency.

Then there is the variety of recombination. The higher the specification (the greater the assembly of sub-assemblies and sub-sub-assemblies), the larger will be the number of discriminable classes.

There are two types of error in recognition, those of inclusion and those of exclusion. Errors of exclusion will become more likely but errors of inclusion will become less likely as we raise sufficiency (reduce tolerance). We may also show that the higher the specification, that is the more information contained in, any combination (as summated at a gate) the lower will be the 'probability' of that configuration and therefore the lower the probability of errors of inclusion, *i.e.* the lower the probability that a random 'noise' configuration will be wrongly recognized. Conversely, where the specification is high, the probability of errors of exclusion is also high but in such a case the risk taken by reducing sufficiency is, for the reason given above, much less. In such cases sufficiency may be reduced considerably and it is safe to accept recognition on the basis of a few highly distinctive clues.

It is my hope that this crude but obvious set of conclusions may incite some statistician to investigate the statistical properties of polyhierarchic connectional networks.

Looking at a single gate with a large number of inputs, it is clear from Pascal's Law that the probability that any configuration will fall within tolerance approaches 0 and 1 asymptotically as we change the sufficiency. When the sufficiency is very near *zero*, the probability is very close to *one*. When the sufficiency is almost *one*, when all inputs must be excited to get an output, the probability of the right configuration of excitation is very small. It approaches *zero* but does not reach it.

Now this is vital. In any system where recognition is a learning process, this asymptotic approach to the 'always' and the 'never' situation is exactly what is required. To the animal before learning, everything is possible. Anything can be anything. As it learns by experience it may become more and more certain but must never be completely so. There must be no lesson so sure that there need be no provision to unlearn it and there must be no mental connection so improbable that it is forever cut off, the opportunity for later reinforcement permanently lost.

I have pointed out that the hierarchic system of summative gates with tolerance is a tolerance accumulator. Sufficiency falls with stratum level. It does so without the disadvantage of the risk of errors of inclusion. The information reaching higher strata has already been filtered. Random or noise configurations have been eliminated at one stage or another as we ascend the strata. Our confidence that we are in the presence of a stimulus which falls within the class boundaries becomes greater and greater as we accumulate more and more evidence from the accumulation of a larger sub-configuration of information from the percept. The polyhierarchic system of decision gates is a semantic filter letting through only what is relevant and excluding the accidental and contingent.

Generalization

I have suggested that, with the growing assurance mentioned above, it may be possible in central regions to reduce sufficiency. The final reduction in sufficiency is that which occurs when some gate somewhere, however many its connections, may be fired or regenerated by any one of them.

This is now fully an 'or' gate and an 'or' gate is a good model of generalization. An org which needs to recognize and act on the appearance of a rabbit would, according to the hypothesis advanced, have to sophisticate many of its internal gates to recognize the various assemblies of the elements of the percept 'rabbit' which might appear to it. It would be greatly helped in its task of recognition, however, if at some central point, one particular gate became an 'or' gate to which all connections which could be excited by the percept 'rabbit' found their way. This process of generalization does not have to happen at one stage and my feeling is that the growing 'orishness' of the more central gates would achieve the effect we require. 'Orish' gates at the centre would enable us very rapidly to reduce the number of loci which are needed to represent a single percept. This is the semantic economy system without which we, as inventors of orgs, could get no further.

Recombination

A restructured version of a percept can be created from the combination of excited generalization gates. We can see an 'old silver spoon with a twisted handle' as an assembly of all the generalized concepts represented by each word of all the 'old', 'silver', 'twisted' etc. It is an 'enough' gate where the generalizations implicit in the description meet.

The Apices

In the central apical region I have suggested must lie the decision centres. To help expositions I have suggested that the apical centres are separated in space and drawn them as though they were particular loci. Within the brain with its hundred million neurons, each of which has a hundred or more dendrites (tentacles) each of which again may have 1,000 connections, synapses, we have an interwoven ramified system of inconceivable complexity. What I am calling gates or loci may be cells but they may also be connected multiplexing systems coextensive with the whole network. They may be cell assemblies as suggested by Hebb. I am deliberately giving a functional description and leaving the neurophysiology to the neurophysiologists. For the purpose of our first crude, rough breadboard model of an invented org, let us pretend for a moment that the org can divide all its perceptions into a limited number of classes, as an insect can. The perception of a complete configuration belonging to one of these classes must be arranged to trigger the 'appropriate' configuration of activity at the motorium. Later, I show that the path of efferent stimulation (instruction signals) must be divergent. One of a limited repertoire of complete activity patterns is to be activated. Just as percepts are built of parts which are built of sub-assemblies which are built of perceptual elements, so motor patterns can be thought of as ascending hierarchies also.

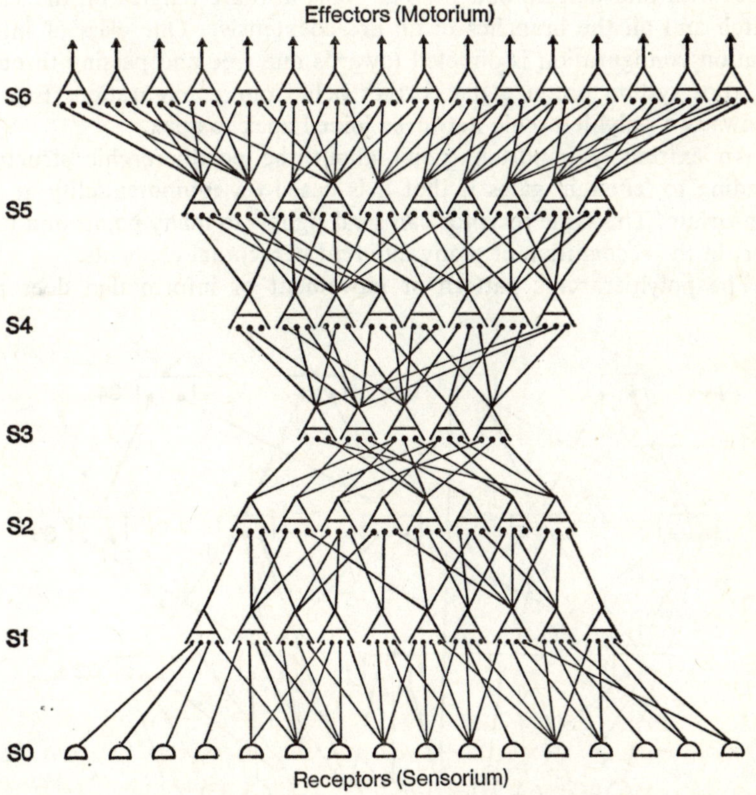

Fig. 17 Two polyhierarchic networks connected at the apices (S3)

Behaviour consists of skills which are composed of sub-skills which are themselves composed of sub-sub-skills. Many of the detailed actions of an insect *pursuing* a prey are much the same as those when the same insect is *being* pursued. It needs to be able to call upon the same sets of detailed leg and wing movements in many cases. The polyhierarchic picture fits as well to the motorium as it does to the sensorium, but here the movement of information is from the apex down towards the motorium as it is in the traditional human organization.

In an organization the supposed pattern is monohierarchic, though, as I think it will be very easy to show when we look at the actual flow of information, the pattern here is polyhierarchic too. As an industrial manager I claim to know. That, in fact, is where I got the idea. The first rough model of the information flow in that mysterious black box, a primitive brain is, then, I suggest, represented by two polyhierarchic structures connected at the apices. It is a root-tree system: there are trees with intertangled boughs. The roots also are tangled on the same patch and all the branches of all are coextensive. One class of information configuration is directed towards one tree and passing through its root system produce the correct behaviour configuration. Fig. 17 shows two polyhierarchic networks joined apex to apex.

An extremely important point about the polyhierarchic structure leading to 'enough' gates is that it is based on equipotentiality at the sensorium. The same receptor can send signals to many points and take part in the recognition of many different perceptual elements.

The polyhierarchic pattern of movement of information does not

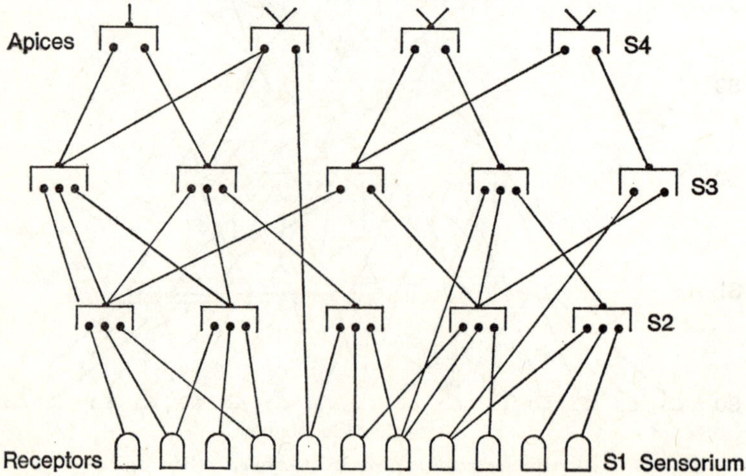

Fig. 18 Connections may skip strata

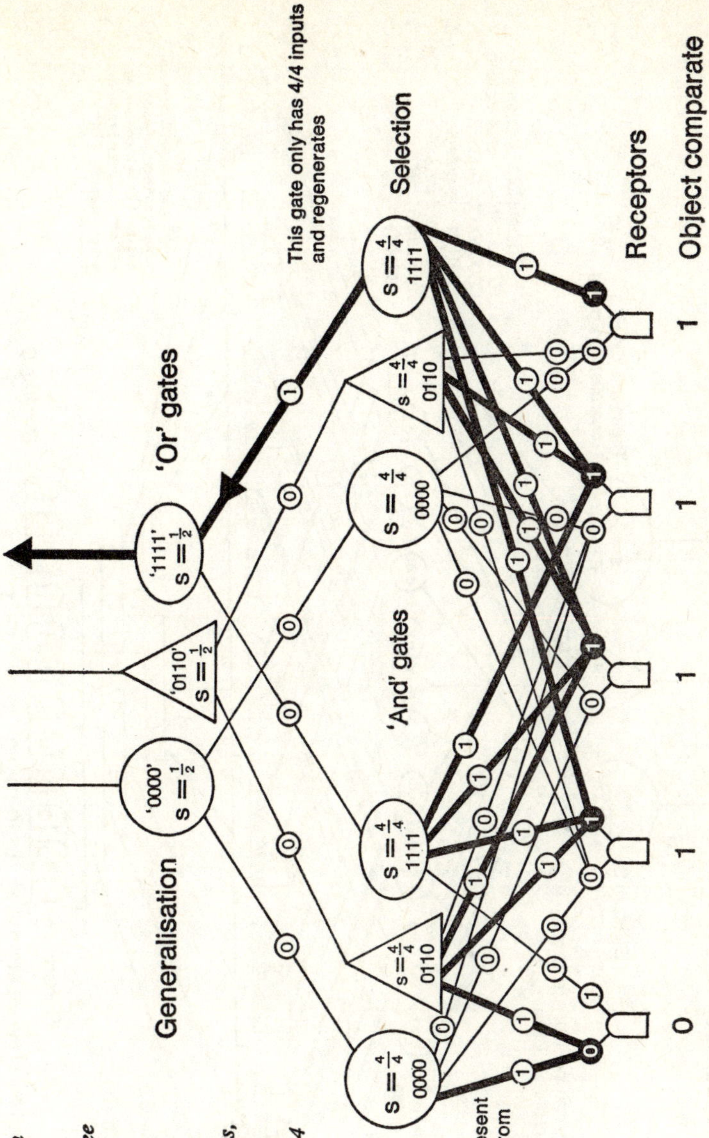

Fig. 19 Discrimination and generalization at three strata. This network can select three of sixteen possible configurations of four inputs at two different positions. At a third stratum they are generalized at 'or' gates, a member of the class '1111' is presented and recognized as it has 4/4 excited inputs

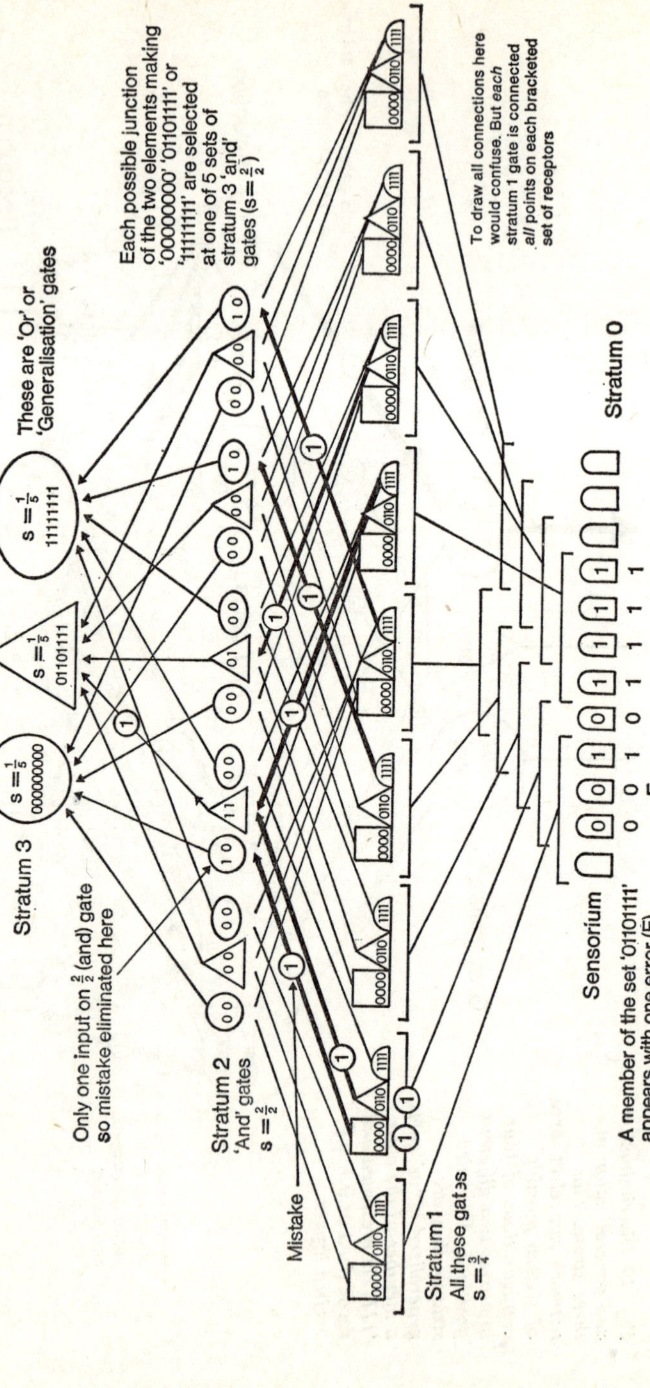

Fig. 20 Recognition regardless of 'register'

preclude the possibility that some signal lines may bypass strata configurations such as that shown in Fig. 18.

We shall need to make more modification to this crude, over simplified picture, but for the purposes of exposition, let us accept it for a moment. There are many things we have not dealt with but the structure may prove to be sufficiently adaptable and explanatory to answer our purpose, it may be an adequate skeleton to bear more flesh.

It is most important to be sure that the polyhierarchic model is fully understood so I add here a few drawings to clarify and help comprehension.

Fig. 19 illustrates discrimination and generalization at three strata regardless of 'register'.

Fig. 20 shows a solution to the 'presentation' or 'register' problem. Three configurations are recognized at a set of loci. The important thing is that the size of the set of possible positions reduces with the number of strata.

The idea that the recognition process has to be a layered, summative, polyhierarchic one first occurred to me in 1956 and I showed a paper based on it to a number of people who signed and dated it at the Philosophy of Science Congress in 1957. One of the predictions I made as a result, which I thought might be taken as confirmation, was that centres might be found in the brain which could be excited only by the appearance of perceptual elements on the retina. At deeper levels I would expect to find centres excited only by more complex forms.

D. H. Hubel and T. N. Wiesel, working on anaesthetized cats, found exactly such effects in 1959. They probed the apical segments of the lateral and post-lateral gyri in the visual area behind the cat's brain. They used tungsten micro-electrodes advanced by a hydraulic positioner. They found cells which had a defined receptive field in the cat's visual field, that is to say, centres which were excited by visual phenomena presented to the cat's eye on a screen. They distinguished two types of ganglion cells, those with 'on' centre, receptive fields and those with 'off' centre fields. They also classified the fields as simple and complex, and there were many kinds. Some cells were excited by black edges, others by lines at various inclinations – the inclinations being always very critical. Complex fields were of many types.

'Two common types of fields . . . each consisting of a narrow elongated area, excitatory or inhibitory, flanked on either side by two regions of the opposite type. In these fields the two flanking regions were symmetrical, *i.e.* they were about equal in area and the responses obtained from them were of about the same magnitude. In addition, there were fields with long narrow centres, excitatory or inhibitory, and asymmetrical flanks . . . for maximum centre response the orientation of the slit was critical, changing the orientation by more than 5 to 10 degrees was usually enough to reduce a response greatly or even abolish it. Moving stimuli were very effective, probably because of the synergistic effects of leaving an inhibitory area and simultaneously entering an excitatory area.'

It seems fairly evident from the above that the process of detecting perceptual elements does occur. Receptive fields varied greatly in size, a quarter to 32 degrees of an arc. Simple fields were at their maximum in number at 2 degrees of an arc. Complex fields reached their maximum between 4 and 8 degrees of an arc. These facts would be consistent with a hypothesis that complex fields were detected when the electrolyte contacted a cell which was a summative centre of a number of simple fields. It follows from the polyhierarchic theory that perceptual elements will generally be smaller than assemblies of them.

Chapter 5 The Motorium

The Apprehension of 'whole situations'

THE PRINCIPAL BUSINESS of the brain in the cell, the animal or the organization is to receive store, code, transduce and utilize incoming information to predict probable future states of the universe and, via those parts of that universe which are under its direct control, its cortex, cytoplasm, if it is a cell its muscles and organs, if an animal, its soldiers, if it is an army, or its workmen if it is a company; to change the state of that external universe in such a way as to increase the probability that it, the org, will continue to *be*. If this is so then its fundamental problem is to sort out relevant information from that which is irrelevant.

If it is the sort of brain which does not know, *ab initio* (as in man) what is significant; it must receive and deal with the largest possible amount of information to start with. Anything *can* have any significance. As I have pointed out this means that it must have many receptors and this reduces the probability that in the complete sense of the word it can ever learn by experience. It cannot learn by experience because it never has any experience twice.

Let us for the purpose of the argument analyse experience into units called 'whole experiences'. A 'whole experience' is any totality of sense impression which is required to trigger a train of behaviour. A whole experience may extend over a second or a year. It is that collection of successively presented configurations which, having been classified, filtered and recombined, add up to the appreciation of a 'whole' situation which requires an action decision. (Leave out of account just now those activities which occur without conscious decision.)

Whole experiences as received are each unique but, as classified and recombined after passing through the mental filters at the lower strata, they do converge at some point or unitary system where they trigger activity. But as I have said we shall need more than externally-generated input to bring the central action triggering gate to sufficiency. We shall need appetitive, proprioceptive and attention inputs also. Once the central gate has reached sufficiency resulting from the reception of enough information (evidence) from the whole sensorium, and this will include the figure and background, both concept and context information, then the final decision is made. The final gate, whatever its physical counterpart may be, cell, cell-assembly or, in the sociological case, committee or person decides; then the trigger is pulled, the switch thrown and the descending hierarchies are activated. The rule of such a gate is, 'if enough afferent then all efferent'. The efferent connections excite their systems and sub-sub-systems.

As we go down we are now producing more outputs than inputs: the component is behaving in the opposite way to a 'gate'.

Let us look at a type of org where we can see it happening. If we tear out conceptually, a commercial firm which, despite the multiplicity of its informational connections with its industrial context, is a usefully separable unit, we shall find that it too has a sensorium and a motorium.

At the input interface it has a multiplicity of receptor points, each of which is a shopkeeper or a salesman equipped with his own complex sensorium. The firm receives each day by telephone, letter, telex and visits, a large and complex array of information, orders, invoices, cheques, enquiries and so on. To deal with this multilinear input and to transduce it into configurations of motor instructions to workmen and suppliers, it has a variety reducing system. It classifies the incoming signals and directs them to specialist reception centres, offices, departments, and so on. Eventually the information reaches a relatively small number of decision centres, planning or ordering offices and moves over on to what is called the 'works' side.

Up to this point, the information has been convergent; from here on, it becomes divergent, moving down through a strata of factories, departments, shops and teams to the motorium or the array of workmen on the floor, each of which, of course has his own extension of this motorium, his own repertoire of highly-specified activities. The flow of the information, which has now become instruction, may move outside the particular firm to its suppliers and through their own information network eventually to an even wider array of workmen in many places.

Theoretically, the information all moves to one centre and all orders issue from it. In practice, if the actual movement of information in any commercial firm (or any other organization for that matter) is examined, it will be found that there is a multiplicity of central decisions, 'gates' (though they may lie within one office), from which elaborate sets of instructions diverge towards the motorium. The commercial firm, once it gets above a certain size, has to classify signals and send them to decision centres which have elaborated efferent information flow systems which transduce the afferent evidential information into efferent instructional information in an appropriate way.

The information is never complete, it is an indeterminate system. It operates when there is *enough* information. Management does not wait for the day which never comes, the day when it knows all. In the case of a commercial firm, the pattern of information flow is patent. My suggestion is that, with a similar interface structure and similar problems the flow of information in the black box 'brain' may follow similar paths.

The flow of information from the planning centres to the works in a firm is definitely polyhierarchic and a polyhierarchic model helps with thinking about brain action also. The only way in which the finite information centre of an organization or the much larger and more complex, but equally finite, human mind can deal with the successive incoming configurations of signals is to put them into classes based on their similarity with each other. Fortunately, the external universe has stable and repetitive aspects and relationships which allow brains to perform their task of analysis and classification sufficiently well to create internal homologous prediction systems after sufficient experience. After it has learned what these relationships are, what are the suitable and viable classes into which experience can be divided, then orgs have simplified their task of defying entropy because they have a built-in predictive system.

Let us consider some implications of our model. I have said that every experience is unique and that classification is impossible unless there is tolerance. Experiences which are *sufficiently* similar to each other are accepted as being members of the same class. This is the fundamental fact of epistemology. We depart from truth or *exact* knowledge at the very moment when we begin to classify. The very words and concepts with which we form our thoughts are distortions and falsifications of reality in respect of the margins of tolerance.

Information

The information obtainable by a brain is always and unavoidably incomplete. It is not given to brains to know the truth. We may know only *enough* truth for some practical purpose, and the truth we know is always associated with the practical purposes we have in mind. The truth of mathematics and logic, it has been argued, is incontrovertible, and it is in that sense that it is redundant. You get out at the end what you put in in the beginning as Goedel spotted. But the fit of any mathematical or logical system to the events in this universe is imperfect and must always be so. For instance, the simple proposition that one plus one equals two can usually be demonstrated with objects. But since no two objects are exactly alike it can be falsified by weighing or measuring and if we choose the wrong object like drops of water one plus one may equal one in some cases and two in others.

H. G. Wells suggested that there is no definition of a chair or 'chairishness' which he could not defeat with the aid of a good carpenter. Let us set an imaginary workman to the task and let him bring us a series of objects which deviate more and more from the norm of the generally accepted class 'chair'. Like the viewing committee at the National Gallery, we might solemnly watch a procession of more and more distorted, but still chairlike, objects paraded before us. At some point, however, we should be shown some odd, mad, distorted artifact which, after a solemn conference, we should decide to exclude forever from the class 'chair'.

Trying to recognize the class; each member of the committee would abstract a particular configuration of signals that fell on his retina from the rest of the visual field. Without conscious purpose he would be paying attention only to that cortical region, for the moment ignoring all else. The selective attention to part of the field is the first step in analysis and it is an essential aspect of classification.

There is, or was, a school of psychologists who advanced the proposition that we recognize objects as a whole. That what we perceive is a *gestalt* (shape) – a total experience. But even the gestalters would agree that figure and background have to be distinguished and this at least is one step in analysis. There are of course a number of subclasses united within the class 'chair' but each of them is understood by analysing it in parts, feet, legs, back, etc. The chair-classifying committee would find itself making analytical decisions such as 'could you sit on it?' 'Has it a back?' 'Has it got legs?'. No one could frame a set of questions, however, such that if, and only if, *all* are answered yes the object is a chair. But conceivable sets of such questions could be asked such that the decision that it was a chair *could* be made if *enough* of the questions were answered positively. So let me define:

> Classification is the process of dividing experiences or elements of experience into classes within which the similarity of the entities concerned is sufficiently great for useful (biologically helpful) predictions to be made.

The chair-judging committee was forced to recognize various parts and aspects of chairs before it was able to see whether the assembly of them was sufficient for the whole chair to be recognized, and the fact of their contiguity, their occurrence in the same place at the same time, is an important part of the process. Something that would be recognized as a chair leg in association with a chair might not be recognized otherwise. The act of recognition always takes places in a context.

At the Cybernetics Congress in Porto Alegre, Brazil in 1972, Heinz von Foerster pointed out to me that dictionaries always work 'the other way round' in defining or explaining a word. They refer upwards to larger classes of lower specification defining a chair as a special piece of furniture rather than in terms of the necessary elements and aspects which make it up. In this sense, dictionaries as aids to the recognition of classes are upside down.

Figure Recognition

The visual appearance of the letter 'a' has connections of some kind with semantic, sonal and vocal motor homologues in the brain. But the written letter 'a' has a number of quite separate forms:

'A' 'a' '*a*'

Each of these requires for its recognition enough of its own particular set of perceptual elements, lines, curves, terminations, spaces. All members of each of these separate classes have to be united at an 'or' gate connection, an 'a' centre which can be excited by any of them. But if we recognize the letter 'a' as part of the word 'has' it may degenerate into a squiggle which would be unrecognizable on its own. But, supported by the contextual evidence of its neighbour letters 'h' and 's' and by the rest of the words in the sentence which make it clear that the word is not 'his', it is recognized. The 'and' gate which summates the sentence does not demand complete, but only enough, evidence. Therefore we may predict that handwriting recognition will never be mechanized without getting up the strata to word recognition. It is interesting to note that work on pattern or figure recognition shows that a multi-layer system is required.

The detection of perceptual elements is also used. One notes the work of Aleksander and Albrow and Parks in this connection.

Working up, as it were, from laboratory practice, these workers are using 'threshold gates' or 'voting gates' which are very close to the 'sufficiency gates' demanded by my purely theoretical thinking.

Chapter 6 **Learning**

To say, at this stage, that my model leaves a lot unexplained, is to make the understatement of the epoch. I have botched up my shaky, tremulous framework and we must now see what happens when we try to fit some of the awkward bits to it. Let us *ad hoc* a bit. Let us say, shall we, that we at least know the general pattern of information movement which we shall require.

In the case of animals with in-built polyhierarchic systems I believe we can sweep the devising of the circuit under the genetic mat and say that, like Topsy, it just growed; but in more advanced animals capable of learning by experience we have to show how an appropriate set of polyhierarchic high-connectivity paths could, as it were, grow as the result of the experiences of the org, its successes and its failures.

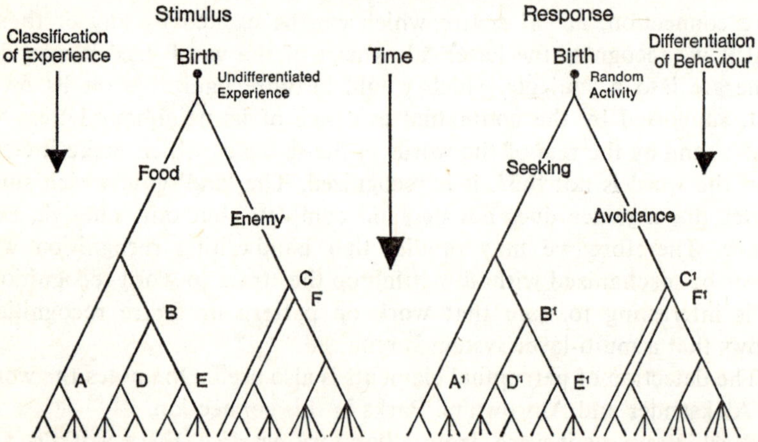

Fig. 21 The differentiation of experience and activity in learning

Fig. 21 illustrates the parallel of the differentiation of experience and behaviour during the development of a complex animal which learns everything afresh at each generation. The sorting and classifying of the experience of events proceeds in parallel with the reduction of randomness in behaviour and the selection of behaviour patterns with ever narrower tolerances and ever proliferating variety. A member of the class of 'whole experiences' B elicits a member of the class of responses B_e: B1 elicits $B1_R$; B2, $B2_R$ and so on. The class boundaries are ever narrowing.

In the sociological case, it is easy to see this happening. As soon as an organization begins to grow, the boss begins to delegate to certain officers, or offices, responsibility for receiving information. The offices each specialize, each receiving a particular kind of information. Those officers on the afferent or input side of the organization – tend to summate and condense their information, and produce a lower number of output signals, which result from the coming together of information from many sources. On the efferent side, beyond the decision centres, the tendency is for instructions to move cascade-wise through stages to a wider and wider number of recipients.

A company receives a large amount of information from many sources, the result of which may be a central decision to manufacture 150 of Line No. 974 mark 3. This is elaborated at a series of stages, until many workmen in the company, and in supplying companies, finally receive instructions which ensure that all the very large number of necessary actions to manufacture the required goods are finally performed.

What we observe could be described in a physiological context as distal reinforcement and lateral inhibition. At the input side of the organization, the tendency for lowered lateral communications between the various centres is often complained of with expressions like 'watertight compartments'. Information receiving officers have little time for each other's concerns, and little interest in them. Their sensitivity is outward to their information sources, and their communication inward towards the decision centres.

There is a popular feeling that you cannot have too much information in an organization, and a tendency to try to spread information in all directions. Too much information is precisely what it is most difficult to avoid. Organization is not the random spreading of information everywhere but the careful direction of highly selected information, limiting its flow so that special attention is paid to that part which is relevant *in each context*. This process consists of eliminating the contingent, fortuitous, unnecessary, peripheral and irrelevant content, i.e. *almost* all of it: not of radiating information everywhere. If too much information is received at any centre the attention to that information which is really relevant is reduced.

The way in which the polyhierarchic pattern of information grows up in the firm does not help us much. Every element in the system is a man with a fully developed polyhierarchic system with its own reward and punishment mechanisms. He can learn by experience which is the most effective way to deal with incoming information and where to send it. The collective experience of the realities of a large information network helps to form it, often without the conscious volition of any one person.

In the physiological case, we have the same problem of filtering out from a great profusion of information the aspects which are relevant and important for the self-preserving activities of the organism. Information must be classified, directed to the appropriate centres, then summated, filtered, and passed on only *if relevant* always *into* the network, and not laterally and confusingly outwards into the lateral sensorium connections. I would expect to find evidence of lateral inhibition, filtering and distal reinforcement in a learning situation. Let us make a model.

Let us take a 3-dimensional region and fill it with tangled, structured, intertwined objects like octopuses. Let this mass of intertwined octopuses grip each other at various points with their tentacles; so that the whole is locked together. We have a connectional or topological system because however much we distort the mass its connections remain the same. Now give each octopus the power in any of its limbs, either to soothe or nip the body or limb of the octopuses it is clutching with its eight legs. It has two kinds of limbs, and as soon as it is excited – it either soothes or nips according to the disposition of that limb. What makes these octopuses get excited? Getting too many nips and not enough soothing. When they are excited they soothe or nip according to the type of tentacle. When they are quiescent, they neither soothe nor nip. Each octopus is an enough-gate which goes into the soothing and nipping routine with its respective legs whenever the amount of nipping it gets exceeds the amount of soothing by more than a certain amount. Nipping is excitation, soothing obviously inhibition.

Now let 'sufficiency', the level of excitability, itself be variable. We have means of calming or exciting the mass generally. Or we may change the threshold of each unit.

Some of the octopuses at one surface of this tangled mass have free tentacles waving in the air – receptors. The world outside is liable to nip these tentacles, and the octopus limb is responsive to this, because it is a receptor specialist. According to how they are set up, the excited octopus will nip and soothe all the neighbours which it has gripped – according to the settings of their limbs. The affected octopuses will go into action if their threshold is exceeded, and providing we have got all the settings right, there will be some generalized excitation moving into the network.

Fig. 22 The building up of a convergent neural link

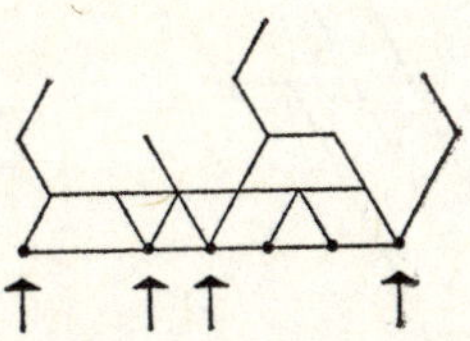

Stage 1 Four signals are received by the network before learning. Plentiful collateral excitation, and a few chance excitation chains extending distally into the network. But a 'significance' signal at all points reduces linkage with gates receiving simultaneous excitation from two sources.

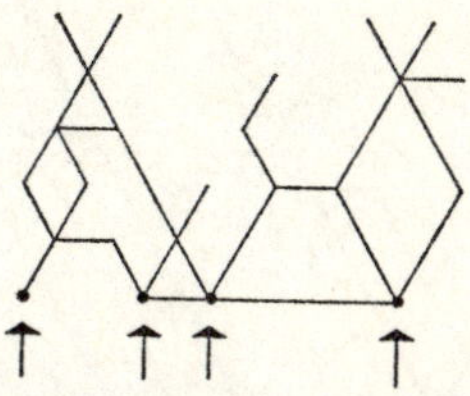

Stage 2 Some of the collateral links are weakened and now fail to pass excitations. Distal links, strengthened, pass excitation deeper into the network. Repeated 'S' signal further strengthens efferent links and weakens collateral links.

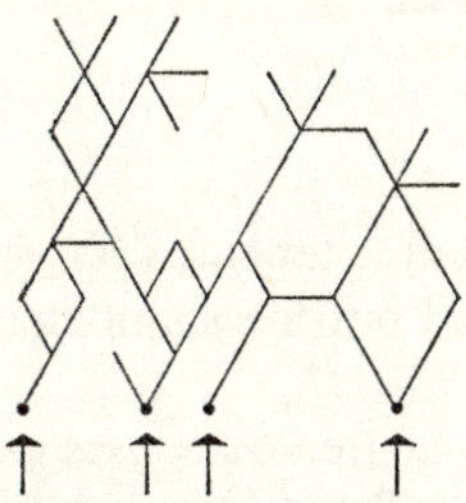

Stage 3 The process continues. Excitation 'searches' deeper into the network for gates of high connectivity with all four gates in the excited nodes. There are now no Stratum 1 collateral links which will excite. 'S' signal repeated.

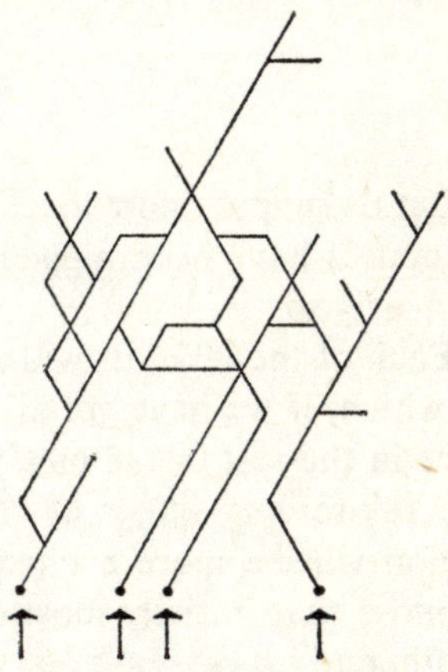

Stage 4 The area of high interaction is pushed further into the network by the collateral inhibition but converges to areas of high connectivity

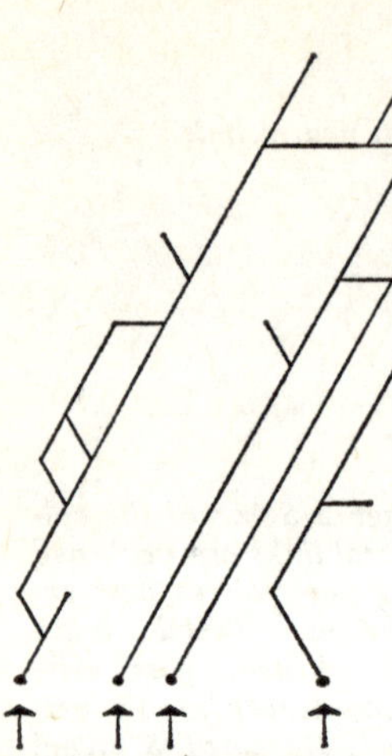

Stage 5 Each line is now nearly isolated. All converge towards the node of maximum interconnectivity.

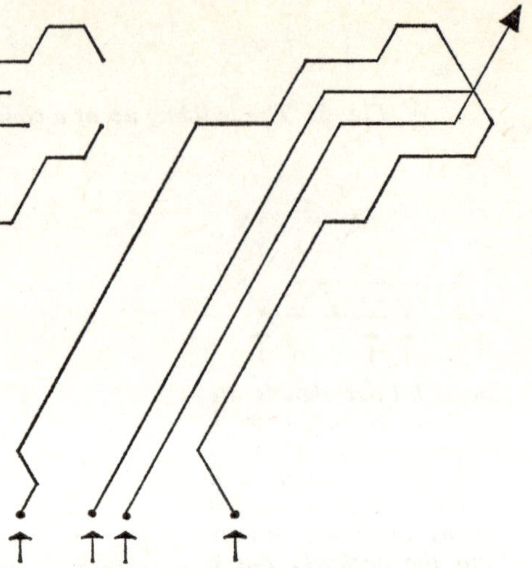

Stage 6 The four lines are now quite isolated and only join up at the node of maximum interconnectivity. Now the summit node only is excited from four of its connections. All of these are efferent, and all collaterals are inhibited.

Let us suppose now that four particular receptor tentacles on various octopuses have been nipped by the harsh world outside simultaneously or nearly so.

Each of these points will develop an aura of excited octopuses around it, which, if we have got all the settings right, will fade out into quiescence in the rest of the messy mass. But somewhere within the network, the reinforcing effect of the four auras will be maximum, and this region will be more excited or more likely to be excited. We have to suppose that initially most of the limbs are nippers and only a few are soothers.

Now let us suppose that we continually repeat the action with the same 4 points. But each time we do it, we lower the threshold or change a few of the octopus limbs from nipping to soothing. We shall eventually reach a situation when it is only the area of the maximum connectivity which is excited when the original 4 receptor tentacles are stimulated. The process of developing a single stage of a hierarchy is one of reduced lateral communication. This is illustrated in Fig. 22.

Introduce another idea: increase the probability of nipping at the distal or far side of the octopus, and increase the probability of soothing laterally. This will improve the effectiveness of this learning process. Of course, if the octopus develops one extremely long tentacle probing much deeper into the network, and if this has a sheath of insulation to prevent it being nipped or soothed by other octopuses on the way, then the tendency is for excitation to move inwards towards the decision centres. The system might work better and this now begins to be more like a brain cell with its 'funnell' of dendrites and 'its sheathed axon'. Now if the mass of tangled octopuses were the brain of an org, we can now see how one hierarchic connection can grow to a state such that only when the 4 particular receptors were simultaneously stimulated, would a single internal point or gate react. Now let us imagine that this particular stimulus of 4 inputs requires a reaction by the org and that another group of seven output octopuses at the far side of the mass are required to nip to start some needed activity. We have now at least a region which will react only to the correct 4 inputs.

How do we build up the right diverging communications to the seven outputs? Initially, the org does not know. It has to find out by trial and error. It has to try different output patterns and change the connection in a different way according to whether they are successful or not.

First, our org inventor will need a device to offer trial arrangements for checking and secondly, it will need a device to measure success. We need a random variation system and a pleasure/pain system. Let there be somewhere within the mass of octopuses a set of them that receives some internal signal, call it hunger, and have got all excited and continue in that state of excitement. And let us imagine that by varying the soothing and nipping behaviour, by the settings of their various limbs, they can influence the direction in the network which a stream of excitement takes. They can play a stream of excitation along the motorium or the levels above it as a fireman may direct a hose up and down the face of a house. Or they can split it into several streams or broaden or narrow the stream. For the moment we shall not ask how they do this.

This set of random *self-starting* octopuses will, if the thresholds are set right, cause sporadic groups of efferent octopuses to be excited. Now the particular group of 7 efferent octopuses which we have posited, must be excited and must have among their random connections, according to the settings of them at some point in the network, a point of maximum connectivity. When this is excited by one particular random output from the central volitional centre it will set at least this particular seven going, or enough of the seven.

Now whenever this happens close in time to a moment when the 4 receptors have successfully fired *their* centre; suppose that some *beneficial* action occurs. Now let us suppose that a further group of octopuses – we may call them a pleasure centre or success-measurer – take note of the beneficial action. If, when this happens, the success-measuring group have the power to send some signals to all octopuses who are at that moment excited, telling them to lower thresholds and/or inhibit lateral communications and increase distal communication – we shall after some repeats achieve a situation in which the maximum connectivity centre of the efferent seven octopuses is the only one which will be excited.

Somewhere within the network also there must be a centre which has the maximum connectivity with the *two* centres we have been discussing. That which maximally connects the afferent 4 tentacles and that which connects the efferent seven tentacles. With the repetition of the 'success' signal and the ubiquitous inhibition of lateral and increase of distal connectivity one common centre between them will soon become the only link. One by one the other links will be eliminated until only this one is left. The system will stop making mistakes and 'get the message'. The tentacle group on the sensorium will have grown a connection to the tentacle group on the motorium.

This ultrasimplistic model of a learning process is a long way from the complications of a stratified polyhierarchic network as described but it is a pointer to show the way. This model shows a simple route which would only serve the very special case described. Where the stimulus consists of an assembly of sensory elements which may occur at any point on the sensorium, a stratified polyhierarchic system would have to be built up at a series of stages. First, the animal would have to be able to recognize any perceptual element, speaking of the retina – short lines at various inclinations, terminations, angles, curves and tiny elements. At the next level, small assemblies of these elements which we recognize, and the next, assemblies of assemblies, and so on, until at the centre be brought together all filtered sensory input necessary to perceive the presence of a whole situation, demanding action.

A mystery that has to be explained is how, in the early stages of the visual sophistication, perceptual elements can be established unrewarded when they represent only part of an experience. Two things help here. One is that the initial power to recognize perceptual elements may be built in. But I have a solution here too, which may be tried out as hardware, see p. 123.

There is evidence that, even in unsophisticated animals which have had no chance to learn to perceive perceptual elements, the means of recognizing them is already in the retina, ready made. The animal has only to learn which assemblies of these elements have significance, either positive or negative, beneficial or hurtful. It is obvious that repetition is part of the learning process that learning is inductive. We now know that we have to 'learn' to see as this hypothesis predicted. There is a stage in the development of a growing child when this learning power is greatest. Those who are born blind but recover their sight in later life (after an operation), find that learning to see is now impossible. The only clue I can offer as to how the facilitation and inhibition process works, how recognition is rewarded even if it brings no biological reward is the following.

If, in some unexpected place, among a crowd of strange faces passing us, we come upon the face of an acquaintance or relative, our face lights up and we are conscious of a warm feeling of pleasure, even if we are not particularly fond of this person. The act of recognition is itself a pleasure. The decision that an entity falls into a known class is an act which gives pleasure in itself. Another way of putting this is to say that experiences which tie in with and do not contradict the general pattern of experience are received with some pleasure, while experiences which jar with and contradict the general trend of experience are greeted with dismay, consternation, annoyance and the initiation of a searching activity as the mind looks for ways to reconcile the new with the old. The searching continues until an 'explanation' is found, a way of fitting the new experience into the old structure becomes apparent and the perceived configuration is at last fitted into the existing classification system. This is a moment of pleasure.

The success and failure registering of an organism operates at its most primitive level in the unfolding of a skilled behaviour pattern. The particular series of activities constituting the whole of a skilled behaviour pattern require to be reinforced very often, at various stages, by some indication of 'success so far'. The success signal acts like an additional input necessary to bring some gate, for the next stage in the behaviour, above sufficiency. What effect do we require the receipt of failure signals to have?

We want to be able to recognize the failure situation so that it can be avoided but we want to be able to separate its centres or loci from the behaviour pattern loci associated with it. So while the needs at the afferent side of the decision apices are the same, recognition, at the efferent side the need is for disconnection. We have to lower the probability that the apex of the hierarchy based on the sensorium will trigger the failure coincident motorium hierarchy. The difference ought to have some physiological representation and we should be able to find in the brains of animals the region where the rules change. The difference between dendrites and axon might be significant. Also, the pyramidal cells, which have more efferent connections and are found in the motor regions, might help the efferent cascade effect we need. In equating the subjective experiences 'pain' and 'pleasure' with 'failure' and 'success' I am open to the usual objection that not all biologically advantageous actions are pleasurable and vice-versa. Some drugs, alcohol and tobacco give pleasure but hurt us, and drawing a festering tooth is painful. But every insentient system, such as the 'rules' or metasystem of a brain, must have a 'balance of advantage' aspect. You cannot make a set of brain working rules which could foresee heroin, something which evidently interferes with the system itself.

Chapter 7 **Attention, Volition, Conation**

Doing one thing at a time

A complex brain which consists of a lot of deterministically connected, root-tree polyhierarchies would never work. There would be no system of priorities. In the presence of a number of stimuli, total situations calling for different and even contradictory activities, it would try to do everything at once and, since all hierarchies lead to the same motorium and need to trigger the same muscles, the associated org would grind to a messy halt or have an epileptic fit.

We have to have a 'one-thing-at-a-time' strategy. In animals we have it. It is called, attention, or volition; attention on the afferent side, volition or conation, intention, set on the efferent side, or at the goal-fixing centre.

How do I add this aspect to the polyhierarchic information flow model; to the multiple root-tree system? Attention is a 'spotlight' playing around the boles of the trees, lighting up one after another. Who holds the torch? The spotlight director is Ego; he is governed by appetites, goals, sub-goals. And he, whatever he is, directs his stream of excitation, his torch beam, according to the balance of a number of forces impinging on him: the appetite balance; the present informational input; the state of arousal (strength of the torch beam); and stored data. There is an internal source of arousal, which sends streams of excitation from lower brain centres towards the central decision apices, selecting first one, then another, for the reinforcing excitation which brings it above threshold to sufficiency, so that it triggers action. In the brain the source of just such an arousal stream is known. It is in the old brain, in the reticular formation.

Fig. 23 illustrates this simply. I have shown a one dimension sensorium and motorium and have made the hierarchical structures simply triangles.

The ancient Arabs thought the liver was the seat of the intellect, the Hebrews said the heart. The Arab says that his friend is the joy of his liver. In the 1936 Harvey Lecture, Penfield said in his lecture on 'the Cerebral Cortex and Consciousness' that there is 'evidence of a level of integration within the central nervous system that is higher than that

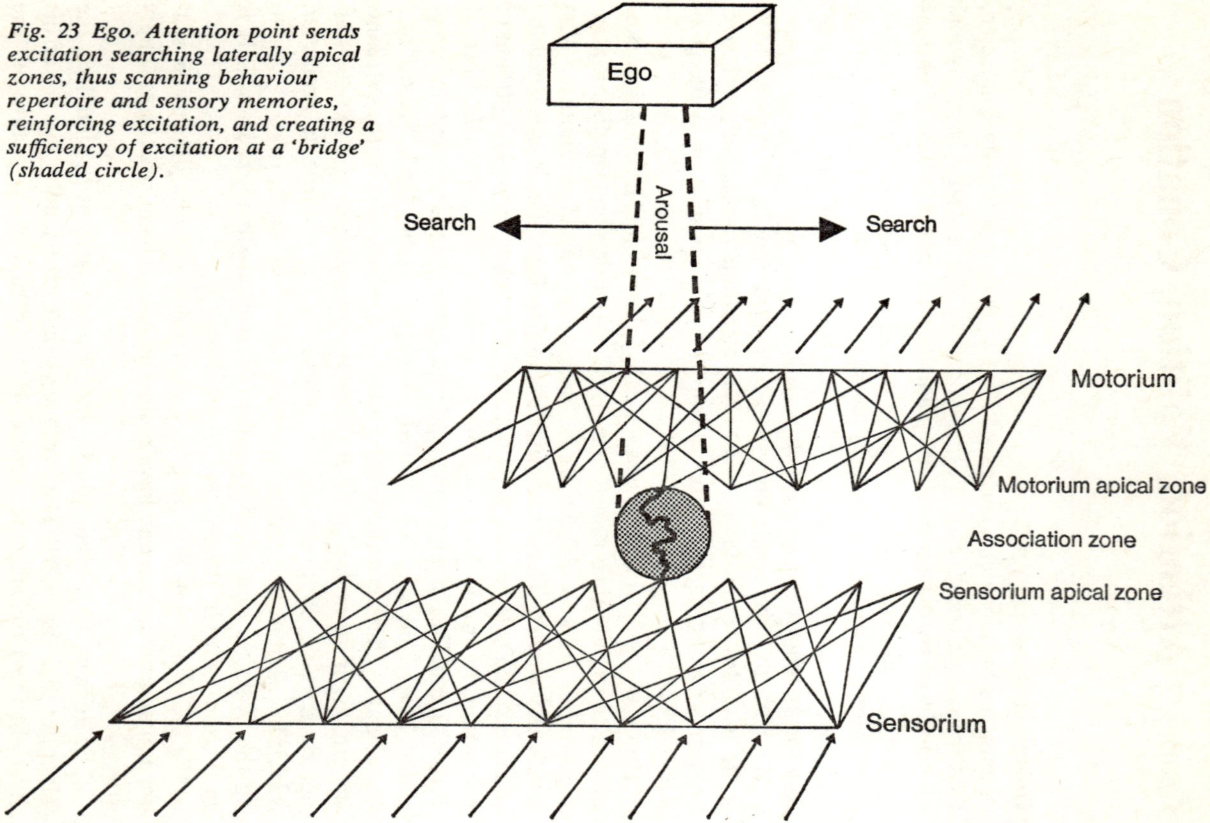

Fig. 23 Ego. Attention point sends excitation searching laterally apical zones, thus scanning behaviour repertoire and sensory memories, reinforcing excitation, and creating a sufficiency of excitation at a 'bridge' (shaded circle).

to be found in the cerebral cortex . . . all regions of the brain *may* well be involved in normal consciousness processes, but the indispensable sub-stratum of consciousness lies outside the cerebral cortex . . . not in the new brain but in the old . . . probably in the diencephalon'.

Hughlings Jackson said that it was in the frontal lobes between the diencephalon and the mesencephalon. Penfield wanted to call it the central integrating region, the centrocephalic system. Sir Herbert Jasper's suggestion as to the function of this, that of 'integrating of varied specific functions from the different parts of one hemisphere'. This was the hypothesis in the early 1950s. Penfield and Roberts point out that this hypothesis has been tested for twenty years by the patients crowding through the Montreal Neurological Institute, 'men and women, conscious and unconscious, with lesions and local epileptic discharges in many different areas, patients seen in the consulting room, in the operating room and also, alas, in the autopsy room. Their experience taken with evidence from many other sources seems to leave no other hypothesis tenable and establishes it as a working theory'.

The picture that emerges is that the new brain is a by-pass or interruption between the input and output lower level apical regions. In a situation where the animal is confronted by contradictory stimuli it begins to think. The stream of excitation seeks among stored data. This can be represented physically by directing a stream of excitation or possibly a number of streams into the area where memory traces have been 'tagged' – that is, along paths among polyhierarchic apices which have a high connectivity, with the various elements representing abstractions or generalizations of what the animal perceived during actual events in its history. The 'tagged' connections would include all the proprioceptive information (which must be treated as afferent information). Thus the presence of the subliminal stream of excitation at a certain spot or region would cause excitation in those loci which represent the highest connectivity with the 'sense of the whole situation' at a certain moment.

These centres, in their turn, would become excited, there would be the possibility of moving the attention region on into them or their ramifications for closer 'examination' or experimental connection. The sensory input of the animal, *at the time* having its effect on the location of the attention point could experimentally 'find' regions associated with the solution of the problem. The search would be like the movement of a spotlight around the central apical region. Each centre that is excited would light up the penumbra of other centres, indicating possible future movements for the ego point itself – like a man who, walking on a dark night with a torch in a wood, throws the light here and there, choosing the next few easiest steps to a place from which he can illuminate another area to take a few more. When the search process brings the moving attention point to the centre of connectivity which summates or connects a successful past experience which may solve the problem, then that centre of the brain has been found, which brings together the particular sensory input at that particular moment and the motor apices leading to what in the past has proved to be appropriate behaviour. Moreover, the stream of central volitional excitation is reaching and reinforcing the same region. This is the *eureka* moment. The animal experiences pleasure. Its doubt becomes certainty. The reinforced excitation is adequate to overcome the threshold releasing the motor hierarchy and set off the appropriate behaviour train.

To give an example there is a baby sitting on a floor and one metre away from it has been placed an unknown object, a coloured box. At this stage there is a set of centres in its brain for 'distinguishable objects'; the baby has an inborn drive to handle, investigate and bite distinguishable objects. The baby has developed a reaching behaviour directed towards such objects. Any part of its visual field which is markedly distinguishable will attract its attention, it will turn its head towards it and focus its eyes upon it. It has slowly learned how to move its hands towards the point which is the focus of its attention. In terms of the hypothesis some centre which might be labelled 'distinguishable unknown object' has been excited and has, for the moment, a connection with some assembly of perceptual elements in the visual field. There may be several distinguishable unknown objects and each has a relatively high probability of attracting the additional excitation from the volitional centre. But the one selected, selected depends upon the previous position of the 'attention' in the network reinforcement which raises the excitation to the point at which the general motive centre 'reach towards centre of attention' is excited. But the reaching fingers can make no contact, send no measurable contact signal. Dissatisfaction is felt and the attention is set into the searching mode again. Among the explorable centres is that which triggers tipping forward and crawling. Among the connections of this centre are memory tags of whole situations in the past where distant objects had been satisfactorily handled after behaviour which could be labelled 'crawling towards the centre of attention'. The child's attention point is now simultaneously at the 'whole situation' centre where the present percepts have the highest connectivity but the stream of excitation from below also brings into excitement another region associated with the past experience of crawling and obtaining an object. These two centres have themselves a centre of highest mutual connectivity and this becomes the bridge which takes the input excitation along the more devious path from 'reaching behaviour' to 'crawl then reach' behaviour. This behaviour is excited and the child reaches the object and experiences the pleasurable feeling of having satisfied its drive to examine its surroundings. The network of connections is reinforced and eventually any example of 'interesting object beyond reach' will almost without volition excite 'crawl then reach' behaviour.

This case does not cover the more sophisticated situation in man where activity may commence suddenly as a result of ratiocination alone in the absence of any sensory input. Here we have to suppose an advanced development by which the volitional, (conative) activity is directed into conative centres associated with sub-goals. We must now suppose that the interplay of the streams of excitation from these centres causes a constant and continuous movement of the attention point, ego, during consciousness, throughout the network in a never-ceasing search for opportunities to fulfil the sub-goals or satisfy the established appetites. Man can have appetites to do many things which do not appear to be biologically advantageous: playing cards or chess, chatting, painting, even writing books.

We might ask why this system of attachment to unbiological sub-goals or offshoots of the appetitive drives has grown up in man.

Men live in complicated societies and groupings. To organize them and keep them going, many types of behaviour are required from many individuals; types of behaviour which are unproductive for that individual except insofar as they bring rewards from society. Certainly, such activities do not bring rewards when they are *new*, until they have established their value. If there had been no random behaviour *without* quick visible fruits and if such behaviour had not been persisted in for long enough for it to pay off socially – in other words, if every member of the primitive societies had behaved at all times with complete selfishness and without attachment to random goals – then complex patterns of social behaviour advantageous to the group but not necessarily to the individual would never have grown up.

But if a division of the evolutionary stream of man had developed in which at least some individuals attached themselves, zealously, to random, personally unprofitable causes . . . then we have the basis of the altruism without which society cannot work. The system has to be experimental. The habit of forming quixotic sub-goals and becoming attached to them with great persistence has to be established without any specification . . . utterly free to experiment, to throw up variations for selection or rejection.

There is no limit whatever to the vast range of human hobbies, interests, games, attachments, habits, loyalties, obsessions. Artists and writers starve in garrets in pursuance of the fierce biologically unadvantageous urge to paint pictures and write poems. Men spend leisure and treasure cultivating dahlias and chrysanthemums, hunting butterflies, hoarding tiny rectangles of perforated paper. You name it, they collect it, do it, love it with persistence and pleasure. Society is thus offered a great range of experimental activities, some of which are bound to be valuable to it in its task of obstinately continuing to be. It is noticeable that this random activity is most intense and various when the individual and the tribe are not under pressure and the life and continuance of the individual and the society is sound. The exploratory search for possible new environments and new exploitations of the given environment becomes more intense in these situations. As with recessive genes in genetics, potentially advantageous change is held in abeyance for chance, better combinations to emerge.

Any system of trial and error, learning by experience, has to have access to indeterminacy at some point. The evident volitional control of the movement of our attention point (region) around the highly interconnected regions of the network is a concept which brings us perilously close to the free will versus determinism controversy.

The one thing that is most patent to us in the universe is that we have the power to direct our attention both actively in inspecting the present state of the real world around and passively in our attention to our previous perceptions or new assemblies of them. All other experience comes from the use of that power; to deny it is to deny all else.

I introduce a kind of indeterminacy within the indeterminacy of our volatile minds. The growth from babyhood of a human being sees the region of indeterminacy being pushed more and more towards the centre. The random input, the experimentalism, is at its maximum at all levels in the baby. Apart from grasping and sucking, we are told, it is born with no established patterns. Its first kicks, jerks, wriggles, shouts, and babbles are random and unproductive, even at the lowest level. Its perception of its surroundings is extremely deficient. It can make no sense of the sensory input. Any input can lead to any output and randomness (or free will) reigns at all levels.

As it grows older it 'learns' or renders more deterministic the networks at the peripheral regions at both the sensorium and the motorium terminals to its knowing and doing. Skills are built up from sub-skills and behaviour patterns are built up from skills. At the other interface, as I believe, perception, too, is built up at first from elements, then from combinations of them, then combinations of combinations, and so on. Once an effective system of analysis and recombination has been established, the org's reaction becomes less and less variable: the probability of connection between input and output higher and higher.

At a later stage in its development the baby plays. Its activity is still largely randomly experimental and exploratory. There is still no immediately beneficial outcome, but it is exploring its environment with more and more sophisticated behaviour patterns and an improved system of detecting what is going on in the world. From both interfaces the randomness is being pushed towards the centre. Free will is the name we give to that little randomness that is left to us once we are adult. Almost all our actions then are obvious, given the state of our appetites, our needs and the perceived opportunities open to us. But in the central region there is still fed in to the system a stream of randomness or indeterminism which can have a major effect on our actions. A man riding a bicycle is behaving like a robot with respect to the overwhelming mass of the information he is receiving with his millions of receptors and the overwhelming mass of detailed instruction he is issuing to each muscle fibre. He is a bicycle-riding machine. His mind is not on the job. His body is receiving the information about the traffic around him, about his state of balance and about his whereabouts and progress without his knowledge and the necessary complicated instructions are given to his muscles. His thoughts are on horse racing or cybernetics. But, on a whim, he may turn up a side road to visit a friend. The system is deterministic at the periphery. Randomness, indeterminacy, acausality has pushed its way up from the tactical region to the strategic and only at that level is the man still free. But to a small boy a bicycle ride is a thing of swoops and swerves, of sudden stops and starts of going 'no hands' and standing on the saddle. His indeterminacy is still at lower strata.

Ratiocination

'Cogito ergo sum.' Descartes, to prove his own existence, had to fall back on the only activity in the universe of which he or any of us could be absolutely sure, his own thoughts. All perceptions may be illusions but the fact of our thoughts cannot be. How does this most central and immediate experience fit into the model? There is thinking which does not express itself in any *behaviour* like speaking or writing. Tired of people like me who insist in trying to poke their blunt and grubby fingers into the black box of the mind, the Skinnerians (I am not sure whether Skinner is one of them) have abolished thinking from the universe. A formidable thought, but *as* a thought unfortunately abolished with the rest. Attempts to understand the connection between the input to a brain and the output from it, on a strictly behaviourist model, have stumbled repeatedly over the insistent obtrusion of this phenomenon of attention in one form or another. Scientists often have to resort to inferential evidence when direct evidence is not available. But to abandon the most direct evidence of all, the *only* direct evidence, in favour of inferences is a strange tactic indeed. Incredibly however, it was in some ways a fruitful one and we must be charitable and accept behaviourism as a 'necessary stage'. Relentlessly pursuing our aim of inventing an org, we have provided it with an attention point which moves around the network triggering action. We have not explained the experimental probings of the network, the devious followings of semantic and relational tracts, the spreading and contracting, the sudden jumps, the pulling together of distant connectivities, the convoluted paths, stops and starts, the dartings and the laboured advances of that central lacing-up system, that palpitating sponge of connections, the centre of our ratiocination. What is it there, wandering round the familiar paths it has made? Whatever it is, it disappears in sleep, is obstructed by alcohol and quickened by some drugs. It can be started by any passing event but, once started, no one can tell where it will stop. Thought is free and being free is unpredictable. We have made so many *ad hoc* additions to our model that we might as well chance another.

Let us imagine a mischievous, curious, exploratory, active, excitable animal, which, by sheer impudence and effrontery has struggled up out of its properly provided ecological niche and, climbing out of this valley over the dangerous hills of exposure, has begun, out of exuberance and adventurousness, to invade the ecological niches of its neighbouring species. The urgency of its curiousity and exploratory drive would land it in some pretty pickles, it would also land it in some quiet and profitable corners. It would have to have a much larger and more varied environment to live in and so its internal records of this would have to be more extensive. It would need a bigger data bank. Its data bank would consist of concepts and percepts, internal subject comparates in the form of generalization gates to which the many classes of percepts had connections. If it had developed an attention system as described, a wandering attention point which could explore its apical regions, it could be rescued from its risky adventuressness by developing a new ability. If a buffer system of loosely coupled connectivity were introduced between the apical centres of perception and the apical centres of motor action; a region of indeterminate and changing connectivity, a barrier between perception and action so that the animal has a means of doing its experimentation within an internal system which is homologous with the external world, it would be able to bring its attention to the firing point behind a motor pattern and hold it there, inactive but latent, while the closely connected regions were explored. In these regions there are concepts and combinations of them which are semantically contiguous, which means inductively connected by many previous coincidences or near coincidences. The animal could explore on an unpunished try-out basis a number of alternative patterns of behaviour and refer to its memory connection for an answer to the question 'what will happen if I do this?'.

I am cheating a little here as I have not dealt with memory yet. I shall do so soon. So let us pass on.

The animal, guess which it is, would seem to have the power to direct its internal attention along any of the association paths, any of the highly probable connections of any part of its renewal network. It may even move down through the strata and look at the detail. The attention zone may occupy the gate for a sentence, the gate for a word or the gate for a letter or the gate for the upright stroke in the 'd'. Just as we can pay attention to one note in a symphony or to any detail of our visual input.

Similarly, the field marshal will talk only to his generals or he may question a brigade commander, company commander, platoon officer, a sergeant in charge of a platoon or even, heaven help us, a soldier.

Memory

And now we must come to memory. If we analyse a moment of memory we can see that it is an assembly of a highly specific group of percepts. The left-behind traces of some past event. Immediate memory is very detailed, with time the details fade. Essentially, remembering is a holding together in attention at one moment of a group of percepts. It is distinguished from an imaginative assembly of percepts or one associated with a plan by the tag 'I have been here before'.

A memory usually concerns a 'unit of experience' with all its contexts and, fitting it to our structure, it could be represented by that point in the connectional network which has the maximum connectivity with all the percepts which were being carried in the mind at the moment, immediately perceived or short-term remembered. It is a point at which the ego's torchlight has rested. We do not remember things to which we did not pay attention. Our explanation of memory must be a chain of points which are highly connected to the high connectivity region of the attention zone as it wanders around the apical cross-reference network under the influence of the ever-changing bombardment of different configurations at the sensorium and the random input from Ego. But like Theseus in the labyrinth at Knossos, the ego marks

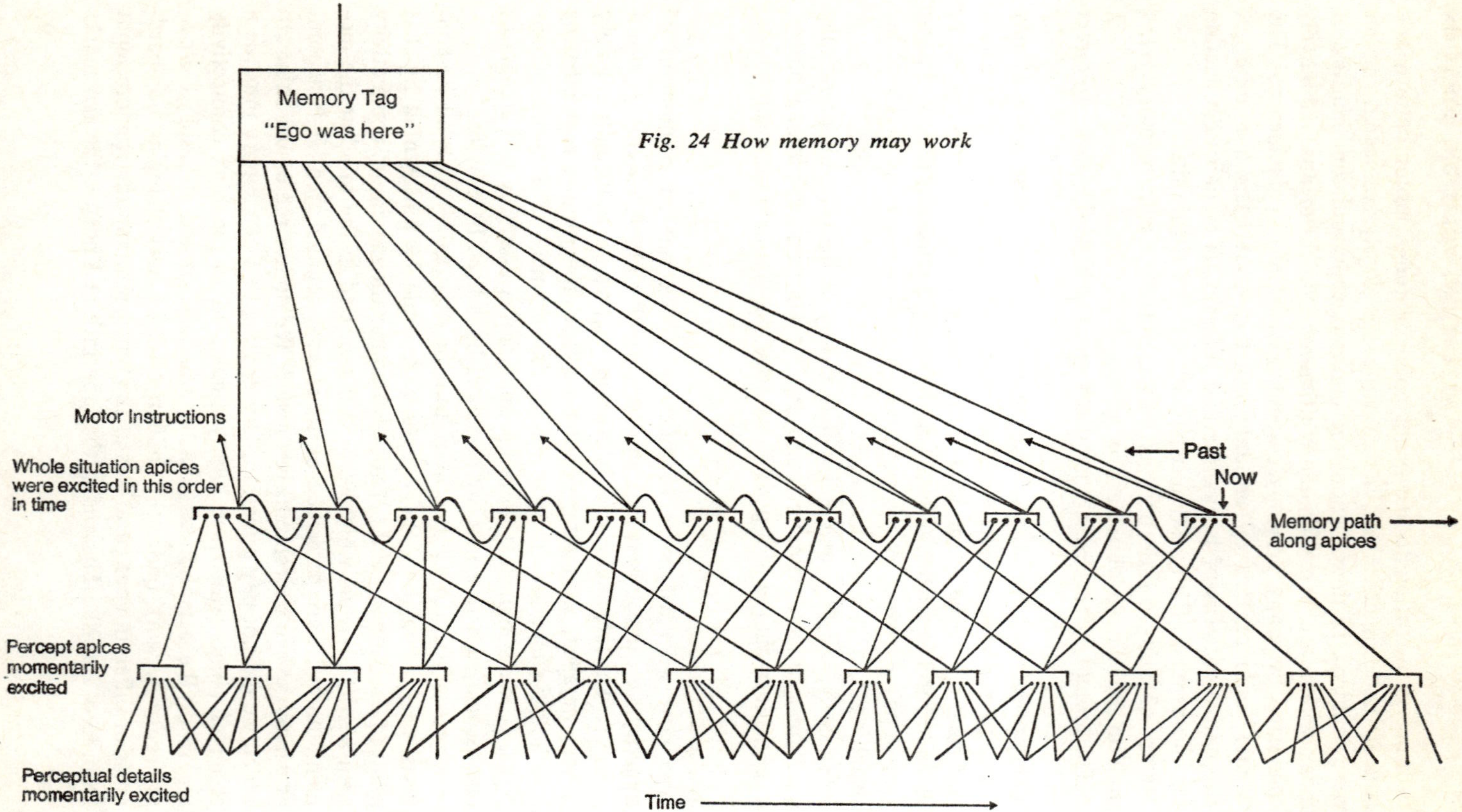

Fig. 24 How memory may work

its path with a string. At each point it leaves a marker, 'Kilroy was here'. One connection with which the *centre* of connections, that class of all classes, the point of highest interconnectivity, never loses touch is that centre which tells where it has been. There is one great 'or' gate. 'This happened.' The idea is illustrated in Fig. 24.

The perception of a 'small silver spoon with a twisted handle' would be the presence of the ego at a point where the connectivity between the perceptual summits representing the generalized ideas 'small', 'spoon', 'twisted', 'handle', 'silver', was maximal. Concepts of such low specification may have many representatives or loci. There will be many points in the brain where the mutual connectivity is high, but at the particular moment of perception there will also be, 'lit up' as it were, a whole contextual background of other concepts coming from other parts of the sensory inputs. The whole system of connections is permanently tagged. An assembly of fantasy and one of memory are distinguished because one is tagged *'déjà vu'* and the other is not. But there is an occasional aberrant phenomenon actually *called 'déjà vu'* where the tag is there but where a number of contra indications convince us that we have *not* been there before. Everything that functions goes wrong sometimes. *But something that does not exist cannot.*

So the presence of the attention point (ego) at a connectivity point uniting a set of loci, each representing an element of the perceived moment, creates a permanent connection with a single centre, the memory centre. Any return of the attention to that point or region will excite the centre which lights the 'memory'.

Electrical stimulation of the surface of the brain in the temporal lobes can produce memories which are extremely precise and detailed. The connective traces appear to be there and the patient is aware that it is a real event that he is remembering. But these kinds of memory experiences are more detailed and precise than normal memory. Apparently unimportant events from childhood are exactly recalled and, what is more, the memory of a past moment continues forward in time while the electrode is applied. In normal memory we can jump backwards and forwards in time or move out along any of the connections to other similar events before or after the one we are remembering.

Imagination would correspond to the movement of the attention point under the compulsion of volitional and sensory forces along paths not tagged as memory points. Imagination ranges from fantasy to concrete planning and is the punishment-free tryout system by which we check the validity and probable usefulness of proposed behaviour patterns.

Now I want to be more precise about my model of the non-active exploration of the connectional patterns in the mind called 'thinking', 'planning', 'imagining' and 'fantasy'. Between the afferent and efferent vertices there is, let us suppose, a large, loosely-connected area or connectional network. In it are 'association pathways' which consist of regions or 'auras' or spreading tentacles of high connectivity (high probability of mutual excitation). These regions are insulated from each other by low connectivity or inhibitive surrounds.

The type of pathway need not be along a single fibre; it is likely to be a multiplexed system of connections. The 'or'-type connection of an array of gates with low probability of excitation operating in parallel can produce a very high probability that some excitation will get through. Neither do the pathways need to be spatially contiguous. Any one path with its multiplex parallel extensions may be co-extensive with the whole network. We shall not expect to be able to interrupt an association pathway by cutting a few strands. But we may find points within the network where excitation may produce startling effects. The whole system may be scanned or searched by a widely ramified but unified system of excitation. This attention excitation proceeds at quite a slow pace in its movement from one cell system to the next. The whole represents a delay or inhibitive system which interposes itself between perception and action. The something, I have called it the 'attention zone', the ramified searching 'lit up' skein is scanning the likely places and bringing together and 'lighting up' the semantic connection of the region it passes through. The search for an optimum efferent pattern for connection to a particular afferent one takes place broadly in a direction parallel to the plane, connectionally speaking, of the set of afferent apices. The final decision gates which trigger action may be thought of as being on the efferent side of the association area we are discussing. As the connectivity centre moves around this region it excites fresh connections and ceases to excite others in regions it has left behind. A man, I repeat the image, moving through a dark and tangled wood at night with a torch, will illuminate an area, find a path, move forward onto it and leave behind in darkness the area previously illuminated. From his new stance, his search will illuminate further pathways and so he progresses through the wood. Similarly I suggest associated centres may be brought into relation, giving the possibility of mutual excitation, as the connectional region, attention, in its wanderings, brings reinforcement. Among the assembly thus activated by additional volitional excitation, may be some already tagged as 'memories' by the previous movement of the attention region.

Planning

What is planning? Confronted by a contradiction, some drive is baulked because some sensory input warns that its fulfilment in a direct way involves threat. A search begins. Some contra-indicating signal raises the threshold of activity and inhibits the obvious action. For example, a child desires a morsel of food and would pick it up, but the food is associated with a hot place, a place the child has learned by experience not to allow his fingers to approach. The conflict sets off the planning mode. The direct action of picking up the food is inhibited, but the volitional flow of excitation is still playing in that region. It is also exciting regions associationally connected with fire, getting things from fire, getting things from fire without burning fingers, and finally reaches the central point which connects all the elements of the behaviour pattern of using a stick to knock morsels of food from fire and waiting until morsel is cool. This has been tagged with the memory tag and is a path between desire and action which bypasses the inhibited 'pick up morsel of food with fingers' connection. An 'and' gate has been found where the inhibitory input is low enough that the additional volitional excitation can bring it above threshold. The associational assemblies brought into relation by the memory tag together with incoming information and the volitional input has sufficient excitatory connections and insufficient inhibitory ones. The balance exceeds some threshold and the behaviour initiating decision gate on the efferent side of the association zone is triggered. Planning is over, a decision has been made and action commences.

In the case of an organization the parallel holds good. The normal inflow of information through sales to the factory occurs in a routine way bypassing the upper management. This is the parallel of autonomic reaction which continues both in the sociological and biological spheres at all times. The phase of conscious 'thought' in the sociological org occurs when unfamiliarity or contradictions cause inhibitions which prevent action and 'higher authority' has to be appealed to. The exploratory phase would be represented by a board room or upper management committee discussion. This may not move physically around the apical regions of the information flow but it could do the equivalent; it could bring to itself those people who represented these particular apices on both the afferent or sales and efferent or works side. Stored information would also be made use of, files consulted as well as those specialists in every organization who do the remembering for everyone. All sorts of patterns of the instruction are discussed, passed in review, and eventually when sufficient evidence had accumulated, all information, a decision is made and the motor hierarchies in that particular organization go into action. Consciousness is an arrangement by which a set of relationships is exposed, 'lit up' and 'held' for a time for examination. The tumbleweed of attention rolls always along regions of high probability, highest connectivity, exposing fresh sets of relationships and leaving behind those it has exposed before.

Talking is also an iterative programme of the same type. The attention, as it were, stepping along the stepping stones of actual words but evoking, as it does so, the relational networks of those words. Talk is composed, phrase by phrase. Each stopping place reveals a new connectional net for the mind to take its next step. In this case the business is going on over the hill in the zone beyond the apices because muscular behaviour, talking, is happening. The attention occupies and excites motor hierarchies with time delays and feedback aids. Sets of words, phrases or sentences are triggered. Probably talking came before planning, for thinking is very like talking to oneself.

Writing

Education by talking and writing are similar. A monolinear string of signals, words, is used to evoke a whole semantic pattern in the mind of the listener or reader. The best writing is multilinear, evocative. The writer has chosen that particular set of words which have an optimum semantic or connective linkage in his mind and therefore probably in the mind of his listener who was brought up in the same world of language and culture. Thus sufficient semantic centres can be excited to light up a 'unit of experience' a 'whole situation requiring action'. The hard work of abstracting and filtering at a multiplicity of strata in the lower hierarchies is bypassed and the information is obtained by the reader in a predigested form ready for action. But the inefficiency of monolinear communication is soon revealed when we try to perform recognition by these means. To recognize someone infallibly by an oral or written description is not easy, even though the describer has chosen the aspects of the person's appearance which are most improbable and thus best differentiate him. When 'sufficient' of these clues have been recited – the long nose, the red hair, the glasses, the stoop – then there is a chance that recognition will occur. But it takes many hundreds of times longer for the recognizer to say 'Harry Jenkins' than he would have done if he just saw him. So speech and writing have the advantage of predigestion but the great disadvantage of monolinearity. We can communicate with each other but not much and not well. If I have communicated no other truth, I hope that this book will convince you of this. It is well adapted to this purpose. My point about verbal recognition is illustrated by a scene from a Marx Brothers movie. A telephone rings, Groucho rushes to it and listens intently:

'That's good!'
'That's good!'
'Oh! that's bad!'
'That's very bad!'
'That's good.'

'What are you doing?' says Beppo.
'Sorting strawberries.'

Chapter 8 **Biomorphic Philosophy**

ONE WAY TO THINK OF PHILOSOPHY is as the meta-system of science; that largely undefined region where the various models and modalities of thinking meet and interact. It is the preliminary model making, exploratory and error-prone probing, which gives rise here and there to sets of concepts or ways of classifying data sufficiently valid, predictive, to permit a new discipline of investigation and to arise and with it a new set of 'laws'.

Another view is that philosophy is concerned with what is out there in the 'external world', and takes for granted the mind itself which is probing it. The biomorphic view which is implicit in Cybernetics approach is at base epistemological. This is the reason for the obsessive interest of those in these indisciplines, with the thinking process itself and with attempts to elaborate hardware which can simulate it.

Epistemology itself is the 'undeveloped country' of philosophy as a discipline, but those, at the other end, the 'hardware' and engineering end of the mental spectrum, those who are investigating artificial intelligence, pattern recognition and biosimulation are engaging in epistemology whether they know it or not. Some scientists feel we can do without philosophy. They think we should just go out there and start looking at nature and finding the regularities and predictive systems that exist all around us. But every investigation has to take place in a framework and he who searches for the truth has at least made the philosophical and ethical decision that 'truth' is a 'good' thing. Also he must classify, before he starts looking for data, otherwise he will stumble, forever lost, through a wilderness of unique events.

You, dear reader, are excessively privileged among the entities in this universe. You are, presumably, human, and we humans, the merest handful of us ($>3<4$ gigaperson), have each been issued with a model of the most complicated, the most highly organized and the most improbable object of which evidence exists in the universe, a human brain. It is philosophically fashionable to create a distinction between that instrument and something which is called 'mind' which is supposed to be quite separate and distinguishable from it. The hypothesis of psycho-physical dualism claims that 'brain', the thing we can look at when we cut open people's heads, and 'mind', the thing we are conscious of directly; are working in unison by coincidence. Since *both* are for all practical purposes 'infinite state machines', the coincidence is infinite and the probability zero. So I shall not trouble with 'mind', but deal with the black box which demonstrably receives all the ingoing information in our material brains and which demonstrably issues instructions to our muscles. The evidence that physical interference with our brains changes our thinking and behaviour is too strong to be ignored. Behavioural science at least establishes that smashed black boxes have zero output.

As I have said earlier, the principal problem with systems which hope to be analogue computers which imitate and predict 'the way things go on out there' is that of knowing which classes of phenomena to look at; how to break the picture up, where to put in the conceptual dissection lines. We falsify as soon as we classify, but we have no alternative and never could have. Philosophical models come from somewhere. Our 'scheme for all there is' is a *model* of some conceptually graspable and verbally transmissible part of 'all there is' and may have to be a very small part of it.

The successive models for philosophy recapitulate the successive modalities of brain function in the development of the baby to the person. The starting point is the solipsist world of a fœtus.

Once born, the baby spends many months in intimate contact with its mother. It feeds from her breasts and is cared for by her hands. As it grows, it lives in a world of experience entirely of human contact. Its whole environment is father, mother, people. Its introduction to inanimate objects is gradual. Its first experience with the inanimate is principally with human artifacts, things made by, used by, and soaked in the smell of, humanity. Only later does it make close acquaintance with things. At this stage it becomes fascinated with objects and artifacts. It acquires toys and is absorbed in them.

But the obsession with inanimate objects gives away at puberty to a new concern, with an intense interest in human relationships and with the roles and structures of the groups within which the developing person is to live. He learns to think of himself as part of various collectivities groups and organizations. He lives, increasingly, in a world of information. He is part of one or more super-beings, orgs, morphostats. His thinking becomes attuned to this. He is not only a living thing. He is part of one or more.

Anthropomorphic philosophies

Following the child's development, the early modalities of human thinking, as civilization developed, were similarly anthropomorphic. The universe was cast in the mould of fathers, mothers, sisters and brothers, amplified into Gods and Devils. The hold of this type of thinking on the human mind is still evident, and most of humanity, even today, can grasp and deal with reality only via the anthropomorphic models set up by the various religions. Montaigne said: 'Man is certainly stark mad! He cannot make a worm yet he will be making gods by dozens'. I am arrogantly trying to make a paper brain for a worm, but I shall forge you no god, so don't expect it.

Mechanomorphic philosophies

Leakey has called us *homo faber*, the tool-making animal. The growing adult is more and more concerned with artifacts, tools, devices. Similarly, as the centuries passed since this sketchy chain of civilizations started a few thousand years ago in Sumer, the tools, artifacts, machines, and industrial activities of man have grown more complex, more reliable and more powerful. Latterly they also became more precise and accurate. It was then that science began. Mankind began to use his tools to explore and measure his environment and himself. The everyday concern of many men became the relatively predictable behaviour of his simple artifacts, and his interest in human relationships became relatively less important. A new style of thinking, of relating mental material, was needed. Bacon, Hobbes, Descartes, began to project a new modality. Instead of seeing the universe of material things in terms of human beings and their relationships, men began to investigate the regularities of experience with the material objects, the tools of science. Thinking began to be mechanomorphic. The world picture was drawn in terms of the interaction of material things. Descartes even reversed the older picture and looked at human beings as mechanisms. Men were seen as elaborate quasi-artifacts. They were material 'objects' which functioned like clockwork (the most elaborate mechanisms known at the time), in mechanical ways. Science used mechanistic models to explain and predict events in the inanimate world and began to turn this style of thinking towards the animate world too. Soon the animists (such as Bergson), those who felt that there was a non-material causality for mental activity were in retreat and the scientific strategy of determinism, of the clockwork universe, was very successful. The assumption of determinism, or strict causality, is that cause and effect are inextricably bound up and that every total state of the universe has one and only one possible succeeding state; one outcome. The advantage of this way of thinking to the scientist was that it prevented him from sweeping under the mat the apparently unpredictable as fundamentally inexplicable. Determinism encouraged the scientist to continue his efforts to explain the irregularities and inconsistencies which he found in his experimental results. The strategy was prodigiously successful. Because of determinist obstinacy, citadel after citadel of ignorance fell to science. The experimental areas where contradiction and uncertainty prevailed were often the most fruitful in producing new and useful knowledge and models.

But all problems were not resolved, though at the turn of the century it looked as though they might be. Only one or two small areas of confusion remained to be cleared up and the God of Strict Causality would reign supreme in a universe which was being run through like a computer programme. There was a messy area to do with the radiation of black bodies. Some confusion about the speed of light. The curious behaviour of certain rare, unimportant kinds of atom which kept flinging a dust of photons in our eyes instead of behaving like the passive structureless units which they were. It would all be cleared up soon.

But it was not cleared up. Physics, the most exact science came all unstuck and messy at the base, the microcosmic level, where it should have been most solid.

Heisenberg, Dirac, Planck faced us with the awkward fact that in the one region where strict causality and determinism had had its greatest successes, there was a substratum of uncertainty which proveably, could never be resolved. Heisenberg showed not only that the more we know about the position of a particle the less we can know about its velocity, and vice-versa, but also, incontrovertibly, that it will never be possible to surmount this particular barrier. Right at its core, the fundamental-particle, the universe exhibited uncertainty or what cannot be distinguished from it, acausality, indeterminism. We can build up near certainty, with large statistical samples, but there is no certainty at the base. We can know, for instance, that particles or photons will be emitted from certain substances at a certain mean rate. We can predict the rate within close limits but no one will ever be able to say how the atoms of the substance decide which particle to emit at which moment.

The determinists were left in a paradoxical position. Their strategy had enabled them to lay the ghosts of many progress-defeating animistic explanations. They had attacked and destroyed many illogical 'faiths'. But in the end they found that the determinism which had been their best tool was itself a 'faith'.

However, mechanomorphic thought, the second modality of philosophy led in astronomy, physics, chemistry to such resounding successes that the exact scientists regard themselves as the aristocracy of Science and often reject the human sciences altogether. Aping the successful strategies, those in the human sciences tried to take over the mechanomorphic modalities which had been so successful for the earlier sciences Psychology, sociology, economics, political science grew up in the shadow of mechanomorphic hypotheses.

Mechanomorphic thinking arises from a meta-system, an epistemological interface between mind and the world in which a very limited number of variables, parameters of variation, are selected and manipulated with all other variables held constant. The initial analysis is made when it emerges that certain isolates from the system give rise to predictive variables which can be measured and recorded. A mathematics which was the obverse of this system arose.

Mathematics is a simple system of symbol manipulation rules in which those patterns of manipulating symbols which happened to fit the way the chosen variables changed, in fact, were chosen and used for prediction. Mathematics had been fruitful enough where a few, say <10 variables are considered. But, human brains have $>10^{10}$ variables. Something else again! Yet the thick cyberneticists go on trying to make mathematical models, ploughing fields with a pin for a ploughshare. Even the micromathematics of a handful of variables working in astronomic, certain, systems had to produce a mathematics of uncertainty, statistics, which arose out of the 'theory of errors' which might have been called the theory of unpredictability. However, the new probablistic mathematics proved to be very useful and made the ineradicable remaining uncertainty at least measurable. The attempts of the social scientists to take over mathematical modalities of thinking brought them more and more into the statistical region of mathematics. Dealing with not a handful of variables, but with great numbers of them; they were unable to control; *all but a few*, as the exact scientist can. What of their efforts?

Mankind on earth today is in the midst of a daunting set of problems. The enlightened are well aware that the only hope for mankind in this age of accelerating and apparently irreversible change, is that the social sciences will begin to create a valid and predictive system. So far they have not been noticeably successful. They have not even solved the basic interface problem, that of recognizing and classifying the isolates with which it is profitable to deal. They are still at the pretaxonomic stage. Psychologists, for instance, have little to show for a century of labour by many, in many places. Some understanding of human and animal behaviour has been achieved; a generation or two has been spent in building up and then dismantling the ways of analysing brain activity put forward by Freud, Jung, Adler. The pioneer psychometrists used and developed statistical methods and were responsible for very important developments in uncertainty techniques and have certainly achieved some success in predicting human intelligence and educability.

But the bulk of the work was done at the beginning of the century and the several generations following in the same disciplines have contented themselves with relatively unsuccessful attempts to dismantle the work of their predecessors.

Marx

In sociology little success is to be seen. The founders of Communism for instance, advanced a 'scientific' method of predicting the behaviour of human beings in the mass. As with every new approach they started at the interface with a new system of classification. Human social behaviour over large areas could be understood and predicted in the framework of simple theoretical models. Laws were proposed which operated like the laws of thermodynamics which relate pressure, volume and temperature in gases in a highly predictive system. A gas is a mass of interacting particles, each of which follows a confused, random, and apparently completely unpredictable path. However, the relationship between the *mass* variables, pressure, temperature and volume, turned out to be highly predictable.

Marx, following Hegel, proclaimed that laws of this type could be applied to the politics of mankind. Despite all the apparently random trends and directions of individual behaviour, the mass outcome was predictable. People could be classified by occupation and social class and these classifications could be related in a system of predictive scientific laws. Though Marx's philosophical and political ideas have gained wide acceptance, his economic predictions have, on the whole, turned out to be not much more valuable than those of astrology.

The assumption that mass action can be predicted breaks down in a world of Maxwell demons, a world of information systems. It depends on the prior assumption that all the elements of a system are equivalent, equiponderous, having equal effect. In systems where there are hierarchies, devices for amplifying indeterminacy, systems in which one element may have a means of affecting the behaviour of many other elements in an expanding, divergent system, laws of mass action do not apply.

So sociologists, political scientists and economists from Marx onwards have shown not the remotest success in predicting any of the sudden storms and tides of activity, opinion and behaviour which have swept across human affairs. No one predicted the hippy, the drop-out, student revolts, the increase in violence, drug-taking and permissiveness or any of the fluctuations of fashion. There have been *post hoc* explanations, but they suffer from the defect described by Popper in the 'Poverty of Historicism'. They cannot be falsified. They can be neither confirmed nor contradicted.

No economist has forecast the tides of economic boom and slump, the excitability of currencies or the apparently random swing of growth and recession. All those in these 'sciences' flounder in a mass of verbiage, producing, as Ginsberg said, vague, verbal, unpredictive models on the one hand, or precise and exact statistical examinations of some trivial detail of a system on the other. They have not produced a hypothesis or law which can pass the first test, that of predicting some improbable, non-trivial event. To compare the work with the exactitude of astronomic prediction or that involved in space travel is to compare a micro pimple with a macro mountain. But it is neither creditable nor, I am afraid, surprising that the exact scientists working confidently in their baby systems among their few simple highly predictive variables are impudent enough to sneer at their brethren with their superman-sized tasks.

But for all that, it is to the social scientists that mankind must turn for salvation, if salvation there is to be. My thesis is that once we see living systems as generators of improbability; once we accept that it is not given to us to be certain; that all we can know are probabilities high or low; we may be able to find a way of understanding the operation of that vast information system, the World Brain, which is already at work, at least autonomically, organizing a World Society. Humanity as a whole is in fact a primitive org, a system which, despite its competitive elements, is in cooperative communication.

Whether the uncertainty which lurks at the foundation of physics and invades the whole of human science is epistemological or natural, pertaining to the interface between mind and the universe or to the universe itself, is a trivial question because, being forever cut off from the answer, we must continue in that knowledge. It is better to know that it will never be possible for the correspondence between what is really there in the universe and what happens in that analogue system, the brain, to be perfect and exact. We are confined, immanently and permanently, to the strategy of the best guess, to trial and error, and to something called judgement which needs a lot more explaining than it has ever had.

Judgement is to do with the weighing of evidence, with making the best decision on the balance of probabilities. Mechanomorphic thinking is a good strategy for making a predictive system of where the operation of a few variables can be isolated. We can investigate the basic building blocks of the physical world with it on the one hand, and the movement of astronomic masses on the other. Determinism is excellent for the macrocosm, has a limited usefulness in the microcosm, but in the 'mesocosm', (neologisms! neologisms!) the human world in between, the world of people, houses, factories, towns, it is just not on. We are forever and permanently confined to balancing the odds.

Making judgements is the process of trying to extract isolates which are 'predictive enough for some purpose' from too great a mass of information and then taking action in the absence of adequate data. The search for certainty is a trap. The best is the enemy of the good. There is no limit to the money, resources and lives that can be wasted if the inexact scientists continue to chase the philosophers stone of certainty. They are better employed in improving guesses and perfecting techniques for recovering quickly from wrong ones. Time is on their side.

Biomorphic thinking

The development of the human sciences, of information theory and cybernetics leads on to a newer modality of human thinking, biomorphic thinking, the kind of thinking that is involved where we have a good manager at the centre of a large organization. He cannot possibly have all the relevant data and he cannot possibly issue detailed instructions to all those affected by his decisions. But, understanding the system, he can guide and lead an immensely complex organization between the rocks and shoals of the many forces which act upon it. Biomorphic thinking corresponds in humanity to the third phase in the development of the growing adult, to thinking in the world of social communication.

Darwin believed that a hypothesis would arise by the rational examination of unselected data. Accumulate enough information he *said*, and by a simple, logical computer-like process, the underlying truth must emerge as a hypothesis. Test the hypothesis by seeing which consequences would falsify it. If you fail to falsify it, it is a law of nature. Another page of the Universal Statute Book has been read.

Darwin's contemporary, Whewell, thinking biomorpically, emphasized the role of judgement or intuition and showed that the real, the important, process was that of forming a hypothesis for test. As Whewell saw it, there was a leap, a sudden recognition, a 'Eureka' moment as Koestler calls it, when a new way of arranging information suddenly becomes clear. The process of collecting data is usually subsequent and is directed to exposing and illustrating what has already been discovered by a puzzling and apparently non-rational semantic leap. We may think of this as the moment when two semantic systems hitherto operating separately in the brain are seen as members of the same class, are united by an 'or'-type gate when the random wanderings of 'attention' bring to an unexpected set of echo connections. This is the moment when the common centre with the greatest connectivity, semantic proximity, is first illuminated by the presence of the ego. It is not a dissimilar moment when the baby discovers that all that class of visual experiences presented by the chocolate drop, in its various presentations, have a unity and a connection with pleasant experiences in the mouth. Recognition is such a familiar part of our lives that we often fail to see how inexplicable it is. Human faces are built on the same plan, yet we can each distinguish with relative infallibility each of many thousands of these closely similar forms. We can see instantly and without doubt that a certain configuration of levels of grey in a photograph is connected with a personality. The moment of recognition is like the moment of discovery. The elements of visual recognition are perceptual elements. The elements of discovery are ideas and concepts. The moment of discovery is the moment when unrelated systems are suddenly seen as a unity. It is perhaps the most exciting and pleasurable moment we can know. To see a friend among strangers, to comprehend a hitherto elusive truth, or to solve a crossword puzzle are for good biological reasons, joys.

The Abnegation of the Intelligentsia

The inadequacies of the mechanomorphic thinking modalities have had the most serious possible consequences; they have led to the rejection by the intellectual of his role and value. There has been an abnegation of responsibility by just that minority of humanity who should feel *most* responsibility; those who, through no virtue in them, have the power to comprehend with less inaccuracy and failure than most; the intelligentsia (I do not apologize for the word).

The successes of science and technology during the Age of Reason and the Age of Technology led to undue expectations that science, 'logic' and 'rationality' would rapidly solve all problems. There are many, even today, who feel that if only all the knowledge could be applied rationally all problems could be solved by simple deductive processes.

What we do *not* know, however, is precisely what is most important. What is not known by the scientist, the politician or the intellectual is how to apply effectively even the knowledge we have. It is the link between sensorium and action apices that is missing. But I will tell you, reader, who *does* know how to change human behaviour: the propagandist, the advertiser and the publicity trade. But they serve sectional interests for short-term and not humanity, for long-term goals. In the capitalist world we have almost been taken over by our artifacts. An attractive but biologically useless product can attract people, buy talent and especially behaviour-changing talent and increase its hold on and control of its human victims. Those who think they are controlling the firms which make these products respond automatically like robots, seeking dividends via sales, via 'created' demand. Who is in charge? Apparently the product itself. *I* would arrogate authority to Man himself, gabby, presumptuous, tricky little beast though he be.

Early in the century, the exuberant scientist and intellectual saw a world in which mankind, freed from the orthodox thought shackles of out-of-date gods and kings would rapidly proceed along ordered logical chains of thought to a Utopia of peace and plenty. Everything would very soon be explained, ordered and predicted. Peace, love and plenty would reign. God was a mathematician and Newton was His Prophet.

Misunderstanding the theory of evolution, Spenser, assumed that evolutionary advance was immanent. Even *within* human societies the principal of the survival of the fittest, would ensure constant progress. Bad arrangements and policies, which were the same thing as non-viable ones, were being eliminated by an ineluctable process, within, as well as between, the boundaries of human societies and organizations. Progress and evolution were the same thing.

But the dream of a smooth and easy climb to an ordered rational world became a nightmare when an uncomprehending generation died in a messy, irrational struggle in the First World War. The war was so senseless and unpredicted that there began a period of disillusion with the human mind and with thinking itself. Rationality had failed, and mind itself seemed to be at fault!

What were the assumptions of the Age of Reason which ended in the traumas of two world wars? Locke, Hume and the utilitarians, following Bacon, Hobbes, Descartes and later Kant, Hegel and Marx, elevated 'Reason', 'Logic', and 'Rationality' – which they saw as a set of mathematical, mechanistic, logical principles – into a system to replace the hard-won treasury of behaviour patterns built up over many thousands of years in cooperating human groups.

The view was that, like the computer (which arose from these modalities), any man, given the same data, must follow the same path to the same conclusions. With proper scientific education, all the bad, old ideas would be cleared away and unanimity must follow automatically. Democracy would ensure that policy would be optimum because all minds, freed from the shackles of old thought-systems, must reach the same conclusions. Kant believed that the mind was so constructed as to follow automatically along logical paths to an understanding of the universe. The underlying nature of the universe was immanent and built in to the human mind. A clockwork mind worked in concert with a clockwork universe.

There is the story of the three scientists, English, French and German, who were set to study a camel. The Frenchman went to the zoo, glanced at a camel and wrote a brilliant and world-shattering 'theory of camels'. The Englishman lived for forty years in the desert and wrote an exhaustive thesis based on his observations which became a standard work. The German retired to his study and evolved the camel from his inner consciousness. Kant was that German.

The intellectuals of the early years of this century came up against the inadequacy of mechanomorphic thinking and, wrongly, became disenchanted with thinking altogether. The Freudians, on the one hand, explained inadequacies by postulating dark hidden forces beneath the mind which control its behaviour, much more than the inflowing pattern of information. The other great school, the Marxist, explained that the errors of thinking arose from class-bias, the sociological pressure of economic forces on the economic molecule, man, outweighing his own rational processes which were still, somehow, contradictorily thought of as chainlike, logical and essentially deterministic. The fact that large numbers of the despised bourgeois accepted Marxist views against the evidence of Marxism seemed to worry no one. The other new view, that which predominates in capitalist societies, the idea that competition is a 'good thing' and that by and large it will 'all work out' if you 'leave well alone' has been discredited even in the parts of the world where it operates. Essentially, it arose from Darwin and Spenser. The error here is that the environment of a world society is not, as conceived, a freely competitive system. It has a single, interlinked communication system and apart from relatively short periods of scattered wars here and there, competition is limited by a very strong system of restraints. The full force of selection cannot operate in a symbiotic environment which is interconnected by one communication system. Competition does not operate fully within one org. And the human race is – very nearly already – one org. An org will protect its parts even if they are not viable themselves in pursuit of its overall aim of stability. Human organizations have governments, leaderships and hierarchical control systems. As Darlington pointed out in *The Evolution of Man in Society*, there is no equivalent to this in a system of unrestrained natural selection.

The Spenserian view that progress equals evolution does not take account of the slow time scale of natural evolution. The recent rapid 'progress', so called, in human societies was, it now seems, the result of an explosion of communications and interaction between many cultural and informational pools and of the amplification of the effect in society of the most intelligent members of it. Industrialism is a device for amplifying intelligence. The thinking of a relatively few skilled, trained and highly intelligent educated people is amplified by a system by which they occupy a role, *i.e.* become a locus or gate in the information system which amplified their intelligence by a polyhierarchic divergent flow of instruction into vast, complex, efficient manufacturing and agricultural systems.

The Spenserian views were rejected by the Liberals and Socialists for the wrong reasons. Though Socialists claimed to be materialists, which means determinists, and to base their thinking on the scientific method, their fundamental moral and political ideas were based on those propagated by Voltaire, Rousseau and the Encyclopaedists. The rights of all human beings were equal and the underlying nature of all men, uncorrupted by institutions, is good and moral. It is the kings, priests and tyrants who have corrupted the world. Withdraw their influence and social cooperation and moral behaviour would be universal. We are still hung up on that set of ideas. Almost all modern politics is based on them. Well, we did away with kings, deposed priests, installed democracy and what happened? It would be idle to pretend that the future of humanity is as assured as it was before we rid ourselves of unchallenged leaders.

But biomorphic thinkers have appeared. Ethologists such as Tinbergen, Lorenz, biologists like Julian Huxley, J. Z. Young, and Medewar, sociologists such as Andreski, geneticists such as Darlington, mathematicians and engineers such as Wiener, cyberneticists such as von Foerster, information theorists such as Shannon, psychologists such as Galton, Burt, Spearman, Terman and Eysenck have begun to probe tentatively into biomorphic modalities of thinking. Darlington defends determinism, but his arguments are pragmatic, not philosophic. As an optimum scientific strategy, determinism had a place. We have no need to defend indeterminism however. Like Churchill's 'difficulties' it will argue for itself. Woe to him that argues against it. Woe to him who forgets that living systems are morphostats, are uncertainty amplifiers, generators of improbability. In the inanimate world, the sum total of the influences on an object is the sum total of its past states and the insignificant uncertainties at the microcosmic level. The whole weight of statistics, the invincible multiplication of probability, drives it along relatively predictable paths to a known state. But morphostats have hooks into the future as well. Their present states can be affected by their predictions of probable future states. In the inanimate world, if we find a trend we can see a direction; predict an outcome. In living systems, the one thing that is certain is that if the morphostat is to continue, the trends will not. At any given moment, every one of the thousands of variables that has to be kept within tolerance, in a living system, is moving towards one or the other of its limits. The safest prediction we can make is that it will not reach them. A trend is *contra-indicative.* Living systems are not trendy, or groovy. They are not going anywhere. They are fluctuating on either side of a norm. To understand them we have to know this and we must remember that our understanding is itself the trigger; the feedback which will help to keep them from following trends to death. It is not true to say that all change is death, but all change other than towards greater changelessness, if taken far enough, is.

Chapter 9 Confirmation and Falsification

IDEAS ARE TWO A PENNY and speculations and hypotheses are in long supply. It is fashionable to say that it is unprofitable and meaningless to advance an hypothesis which cannot be falsified. I am not sure that I adhere to this extreme view. As I have said elsewhere, just as the anthropomorphic system of gods and devils may have had a biological value unconnected with its semantic content, so there may be stateable but unfalsifiable propositions that relate experience usefully and present a conceptual arrangement which aids the mind in its work and helps it to 'grasp' encoded reality; helps it at the interface where reality is being classified and before propositions about classes have been formulated.

However, the set of loosely connected hypotheses that I have put forward are by no means untestable. There is evidence which is compatible with them and other evidence which is not so. When I first advanced the suggestion that the flow of information into and out of a brain could be understood as two polyhierarchic structures, afferent and efferent, connected at the two sets of apices, I made a number of predictions which would follow from it. I showed a paper about it to several people at the Philosophy of Science Congress in 1957. They included Ross Ashby, Professor Kapp and others. The paper was read, signed and dated. Later in a paper for the *Scientist Speculates* I wrote about 10,000 words expanding my original theme. This was condensed by Professor John Good into a very short piece in the book, with references to papers I had never seen. In the second paper, I made a number of predictions which would be confirmatory of my hypothesis. And the weight of confirmation has grown heavy. However, some things are so obvious that the experiment to confirm them sounds ridiculous.

Take my thesis that the principal underlying aspect of living systems is morphostasis, a proposition that I have advanced to many audiences without, as far as I can remember, ever finding much agreement. Experiments to prove that living things behave as time-defying systems, that it is legitimate to classify them as morphostats, are almost too easy to devise. We could take a large, matched sample of dogs, or if we are afraid of unpopularity, politicians, put them in a chamber, reduce the air supply until half are asphyxiated. We then subject them both to revival procedure and keep both the dead ones and the lives ones together in exactly the same environment, providing both with the same food and water for a six-month period observing both at intervals. Measurement would be taken of the chemical condition, shape, size, mobility, heart rate, pulse, blood salinity of the animal and of the corpses with a careful note being made of any deviations from norm of any of these parameters. I predict that it would soon become clear that the group that passed, by whatever tiny margin, the asphyxia point and died would go through morphological changes which would be quantitatively different from those occurring to the living group. I even think that the differences would have statistical significance. It would also be evident on experiment that those whose brains were still functioning would be coextensive with the 'stable' group. The hypothesis is not falsified and my prediction would come true. My thesis that the principal activity of a brain is to ensure morphostasis, is more difficult to falsify because a single example of an action which is not biologically advantageous would not disprove the proposition and it would rarely be possible to say whether an action which is non-morphostatic at one level may be morphostatic at another. Phylogenetic disadvantages may be ontogenetic advantages. Experimentalism and the exploratory drive create difficulty because only a small proportion of the activity may pay off biologically and yet it may still be worthwhile. The only experiment I can suggest is to breed two populations of wild animals apart, on the basis of their propensity for being exploratory; developing two strains, 'explorers' and 'incurious'. Three populations including 'normals' would then be released into a wild environment and I predict that the explorers and the 'incurious' would be eliminated and the normal wild animal with the normal level of exploratory drive and curiosity only would survive. This would be evidence that a proper level of experimentalism is morphostatic.

The Model and the Difficulties

I want to show how the model proposed helps with some of the difficulties that have to be solved by any model of mental action. The first difficulty is the lack of a one-to-one relationship between input and output; it is concerned with explaining the autonomous internal contribution to the mental processes. My solution is to accept that there must be some autonomous central processes corresponding to arousal, to appetites, their satisfaction and its measurement. Memory I explain as an 'or' gate connection of many centres to a 'memory centre'. The delay between stimulus and response has been given no physical explanation but the need for delay, while searching and cross-relating proceed is shown. The posited searching activity of the arousal stream might provide a suitable model. There is need for some internal clock also to give timing signals for rhythmic behaviour and timed behaviour. The polyhierarchic hypothesis is clearly a connectional one and models of this type present many difficulties. In my model, however, percepts of low specification would have many loci and percepts or concepts of high specification are not likely to be missed. This would explain why cortical excision has little effect or can be overcome in time.

The apparently spontaneous firing of neurons is required to supply the random input necessary for learning.

The closed self-reinforcing circuits discovered by Lashley in the cortex are no problem and simply help with short-term memory. The fact that learned discrimination does not appear to depend on particular cells can be explained by multiplexing, but, as Hubel and Wiesel showed there are particular cells with special discriminative functions at low strata.

Generalization

Generalization can be explained by an 'or' type connection to a gate.

Equipotentiality, explains the fact that different stimuli can arouse the same responses (tolerance) or that it does not matter what sensory cells are excited in order to get a certain response. This is required for the hypothesis.

Polyak showed that the same shape would give different cortical projections, on different parts of the eye.

These differences are constant for any particular area of the cortex so the 'perceptual element detectors' in a distorted area would correct that distortion. From the point of view of the receptors in a peripheral distorted area, *i.e.* a curved line might be interpreted as straight if the curvature was due to optical factors.

The instability of attention is accounted for as the hypothesis posits that attention shall be at least partially exploratory in function. Attention has three inputs, appetite, perception and randomness. Its direction is decided by the balance.

The great tolerance of biological recognition is explained by the fact that tolerance is cumulative in ascending strata.

The vast number of classes of events that can be distinguished perceptually is not difficult to explain on a system in which there is no limit to the number of hierarchical communication structures which can be built on the same base.

A Confirmatory Experiment

How is the network somewhere behind the visual cortex taught to see by this hypothesis? Many apical gates must be programmed, one for each set of perceptual elements.

I have done some experimental work on this and can report the results. I was in my laboratory, the World, the other day, when I turned those sophisticated visual class discriminating instruments, my eyes, on to a baby in the act of learning to know and to know how to deal with that class of entities the generalization loci of which I can excite in your brain by using the words 'chocolate drop'.

I produced a strange object and the baby's incessant random exploratory movements stopped and his eyes focused on this strange new entity that had swum into his receptive field, his ken. With some apparent difficulty and not without mistakes he brought those unfamiliar instruments, his hands, to bear upon the task of getting the entity into his control. He then held it up and, as well as he could for his lack of skill, turned it over, twisted it, moved it around and studied it closely for over a minute. Every part of his retina was receiving many images in rapid succession. Then he transferred it to his mouth and explored it with his lips and tongue before it disappeared. A second chocolate drop produced a similar reaction but, the inspection time-span was shorter. On the presentation of the third chocolate drop the exploratory phase was already much diminished. Within ten minutes it was evident that I had, at least, temporarily, while the appetite lasted, created a chocolate-eating automaton. Every appearance of the stimulus was rapidly followed by the immediate and identical response. What had happened? One particular exploratory effort for the baby was paid off. The baby has learned to know the chocolate drop as a phenomenon and he learned to know it before he was rewarded. In quick succession he presented all parts of his retina with stimulation in the form of those elements and assemblies which make up a chocolate drop in its various presentations. Its brownness, its curves and planes, its feel, its smell and taste were successively and slowly experienced. Messages from widely separated and very different sensory instruments found their way together to trigger an automatic response for a period of many minutes. The connection, or set of them, was made, ready to be activated at any time in the future when the appetite for the sweet things should be strong and the attention suitably directed. The child had not only learned about the class 'chocolate drop', its uses and advantages; it had learned to see it. At some later stage he will learn to connect it with motor patterns other than the 'grab and eat' response, he will learn to say and later to write the encoded symbolic sounds and marks on paper which will help him to bring the attention of other people to this class of entity and he will be rewarded with chocolate drops for his effort. For the rest of his life he will be able to evoke the idea at will and the semantic connection system attached to it will grow and elaborate. He will learn that 'chocolate drop' is a sub-set of the set 'sweets' of the set 'chocolates' of the set 'food' of the set 'brown things' and so on, almost *ad finitum*. But not quite.

Hardware for Testing the Hypothesis

Dear old Poppa Popper says you cannot prove anything. You can only disprove it. If you go on trying to disprove it long enough and fail then, and only then, may you provisionally accept it while waiting for your scientific successor to chop you up. This is very nice for paid academic meditators and true enough because it is not given to brains to be *certain*, but it is also trivial; not much use to an org which has to predict in a world of uncertainty and therefore has to decide what evidence is sufficient – always. So, though 'you don't chop your poppa up in Massachusetts', I shall have to do so here.

Orgs must predict to survive. They have no basis for prediction except experience. Experience is induction. Nothing else can be retained. Brain is an inductive machine which filters the repetitive from the ephemeral. Popper dismissed induction from philosophy saying that nothing need be said about it. Since brains have no grip on anything but the repeatability of phenomena, I feel he was rash.

Do not, please, you hardy few survivors of my readers, do not be taken in by all that guff about the 'truth' of the axiomatic systems of mathematics.

They say that you set them up to be self-consistent and therefore by definition they are 'true'. True! *Schmue*! True but useless. There is an infinity of axiomatic systems which the crazy human mind could invent but only a handful of them happen to be a rough fit to the way bits of nature go on outside of us. What mathematicians forget is the survival of the fittest among mathematical theories (or, ways of manipulating a handful of symbols). We are only looking at the survivors. There is no magic about it, simply a restatement of the old truths that what works, works; what survives, survives. Sure enough, odd bits of mathematical curiosity sometimes lay around for years and were later found to fit somewhere. 'Look. God is a mathematician,' says the mathematician, 'see what mathematics foresaw.' Rubbish! there is no foreseeing until we look at the whole set of mathematical theories, including the screwed up pieces of paper from the wastepaper baskets. What proportion chanced to to be useful? Some did because they were modelled on 'what is going on out there'. They were a deliberate attempt to ape it. But the 'pure' mathematician is playing games, making many models and leaving the applied mathematician to pick out the good 'uns. It would be odd if some of them did *not* fit the universe, here and there, by and large, with more or less tolerance. So the internal 'truth' of mathematics is a different 'truth', semantically, from the other meaning of 'truth' which is a fit to what goes on out there. From Goedel's Theorem we see that mathematics is a shop. If you go in with nothing, you come out with nothing. If you go in with money, information about the universe, you may buy transduced, transformed and more useful and predictive information. But nothing is for nothing, nothing is for free. Kant was wrong, and you get nothing out of mathematics you do not put in. So these 'rules of logic' and 'rules of deduction' are merely a widely applicable selection from lots of other sets of rules and I firmly say:

'The rules of deduction were inductively apprehended.'

Brain learned, by repeated experience, which logical processes worked out best and we slung aside a pile of rejects which did not. Poppa Popper, incidentally, gave the best Mensa Annual Lecture we ever had, making the stern condition no one of his delighted audience of 400 be allowed to sneak a single drag at a fag. He is a lovely man, God bless him, but wrong to hell in the opinion of this particular over-promoted woodworking machinist. Popper denies me confirmation but I would like to prove my hypothesis. He sets me, a very busy man, the task of spending years trying to disprove it. I am sorry I am too busy. I believe it is the other way round. We living people, who have to make our way in the world and produce goods and services for each other and for philosophers, and scientists, we have to chance it and work on something called evidence, on the balance of probabilities. There *is* such a thing as evidence. It works like this. Set up a hypothesis, a model or scheme you claim to have some kind of 'fit' with 'what goes on out there' in the external universe. Try to calculate the consequences of your hypothesis and make a prediction, as unexpected as possible, from it. The lower the probability appears to be, before you start, that your prediction will be fulfilled, the stronger the evidence if it is. The concept, '*a priori* probability' is tricky I admit, but it means what are the chances against a 'chance explanation'? The higher these are the stronger the evidence. That is the basis of the concept of statistical significance and what we do with a χ^2 test. But the type of connectional models I have made to give the opportunity to ascribe an *a priori* probability to a class of events or percepts. The probability of

the class 'orange', for instance, is the reciprocal of the total variety of objects perceivable by the sensorium concerned divided by the 'band-width' or sufficiency of the presentation of members of the class 'orange' to the sensorium
i.e.:

$$Po = \frac{Var\ S_o}{Var_n}$$

Where Po = the a priori probability of the entity 'orange' Var S_o = the variety of presentations of 'orange' within the sufficiency of that class and Var_n = the variety of possible visible configurations for the sensorium concerned (approximately 2^n where n receptors are concerned).

One test of my hypothesis would be if a polyhierarchic connectional network, such as I have described, be built as 'hardware' if we found that, by and large, it worked. Any reader with a few megadollars to spare will have my full backing in this experiment.

The little bit of the problem which with friends I am trying to sort out is:

What kind of 'component' would be needed to do the job of the 'octopuses' I mentioned earlier. We might as well admit it, we are trying to make a model of a neuron and, based on the hypothesis we are trying to make, one that will 'learn' to discriminate pattern by being rewarded and punished. We are trying to figure out how to ask a computer, what the rules have to be for the connections between the components must be, what kind of program they must have, what kind of inputs and so on. The general hypothesis is that a neuron is a 'gate' and can change between being an 'and' gate and an 'or' gate. My speculations have led me to a rough idea of a design, for the gate needed. I asked the people who had been working in the field of pattern recognition and I found that a similar component had been developed. I was working down from the theory and they were playing about with hardware trying to make it recognize pattern.

I called mine a 'sufficiency' gate, a gate which regenerates when a number of its excitatory inputs exceeds the number of its inhibitory inputs by a 'sufficient' amount. Other names for this component, independently invented in various places where pattern recognition work is going on, are 'voting gate' and 'threshold gate'.

In what follows I am trying to probe a little farther and show a primitive model of a self-programming, learning, gate which would lead to the kind of polyhierarchic information flow in a neural network which I have posited.

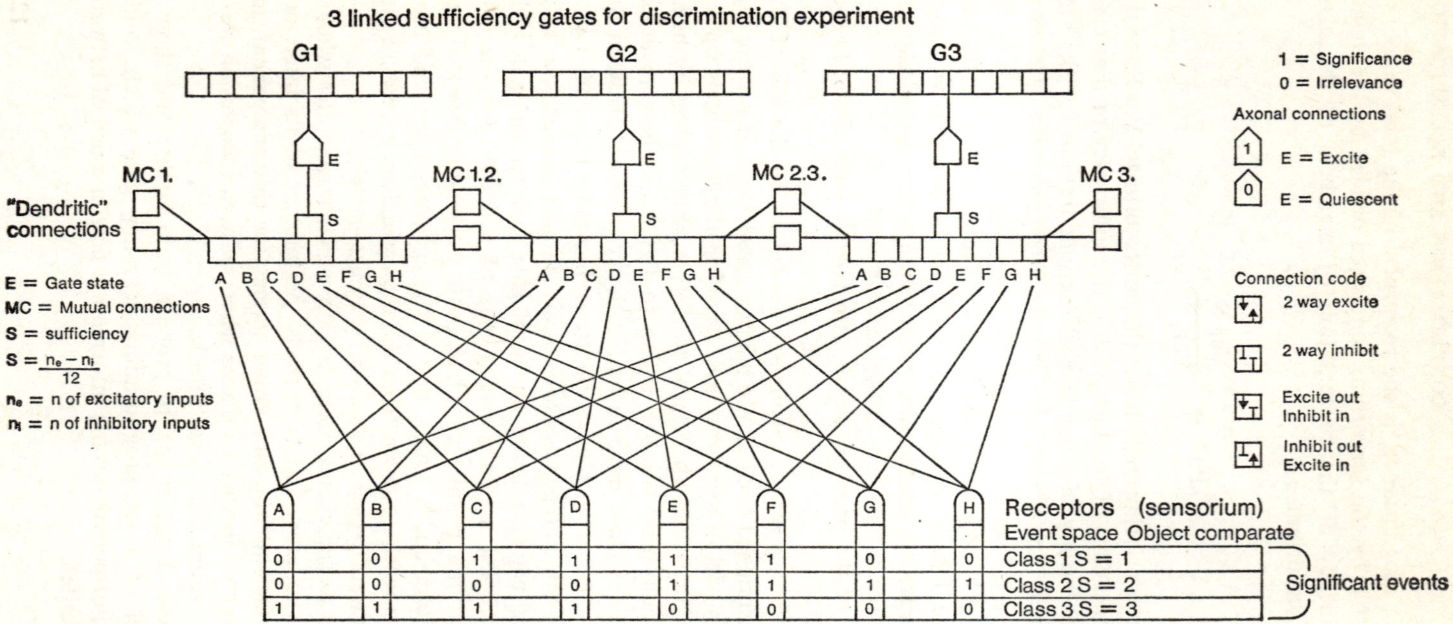

A	B	C	D	E	F	G	H	
0	0	1	1	1	1	0	0	Class 1 S = 1
0	0	0	0	1	1	1	1	Class 2 S = 2
1	1	1	1	0	0	0	0	Class 3 S = 3

Fig. 25 Model of nerve cell programming

In Fig. 25 we see the sensorium, an array of receptors and below them, set out conveniently, the classes of event that can occur in the limited universe of this org. These three events '0011100' and '00001111' and '11110000' have different 'significance' for the org. We do not care at this stage whether 'good' or 'bad'. It has to learn to know both kinds. In real life, we are allowed as many gates as we like, ten million of them, each with about a hundred inputs of tentacles (dendrites) and with the long or short axon probing into the network and having a diverging 'river delta' at the far end of output connection. We know already that it is 'summative' in that it fires if enough of its inputs fire. This is exactly what we need. In the diagram I have given my poor little gates only eight dendrites. If we think of these as the lines connecting A-A, B-B, C-C, you will see that all three gates are looking at the same set of receptors. I do not show more to avoid confusion. They also have interconnections, the boxes marked MC and the other boxes marked dendritic connections are program boxes. In the cell they are called synapses. They receive instructions about what to do with an incoming signal, whether to make it excitatory or inhibitory, whether to count up or count down, whether to be indicative or contra-indicative. In the boxes marked S we may put a fraction from $\frac{1}{12}$: then the gate is an 'or' gate and will respond to any of its twelve inputs. When S = 12/12, when it insists on all its inputs being 'confirmatory' before it will fire, it is a full 'and' gate, a bloody fussy gate. This quality, 'sufficiency' or fussiness, is a variable of the learning process. In the little arrow-shaped box above E we may write 1 if the cell excites, or 0 if it does not. At the top we have another row of boxes giving the places where we write the output program. Each box contains some instruction like 'if cell fires send inhibition'; 'if the cell fires do nothing' or 'send excitation'.

The program is variable and, this is quite essential, variable by chance. In the computer we shall have to apply to a table of random numbers to find out what the first settings are to be. This is not so of the S box settings. They are set lowish. We shall have to have something else to give this instructions to the program boxes. We shall need a 'metaprogram', a 'ubiquitous signal', to instruct the program boxes when to change randomly and when not to. This 'ubiquitous' signal seems likely to operate only on activated boxes. It is important to note that there is no reason why a synaptic box should not be inhibitory in one direction and excitatory in the other. In fact, I rather think it may have to be. The role of the gate is as before: 'if enough afferent then all efferent'. If 'fire' then 'carry out instructions'. Now the metaprogram is set to operate on the 'success' or 'failure' signal without which we cannot do any learning. At the sensorium end, success and failure are both 'significant'. The event, whatever it was, is one of those events which are important to the organism, one upon which it may need to act. At the distal, axonal end, there will be a differential effect from the 'success' and 'failure' because we have to cut down connections with 'bad' behaviour hierarchies and try to search for better ones.

Let us think of the dendritic end first. Three gates are looking at an empty space called 'event space'. The reader can play the game. Xerox off a few copies and try. Apply to a table of random numbers and set the dendritic and mutual connections on some rule you have preformulated so that the table of random numbers tells you what to do. You mustn't alter the instructions as you go, you should start the experiment anew if it does not work. All we are allowed to know is whether significance is achieved in one or more of the boxes fired. Now start our universe up. With another preset rule, ask the random number table or throw dice to decide which events in turn are to be lifted into the 'event' space.

With this random setup, some boxes counting up and some counting down, when an event comes up there is likely to be one box which has got a better match, therefore a higher score, E-I where E = excitatory inputs and I = inhibitory inputs, that are activated. Sufficiency is set low to start with as what we are doing is setting up a competition to try and get the gates to 'home in' on discrimination. Maybe at the first shot we get all three gates to fire, all receive sufficient excitation. My thesis is that there is a set of rules which will cause the three gates to learn to specialize in a particular percept or event class. The kind of rule change, the metaprogram which would then apply to the dendritic program boxes is something like this. At each excitatory input on a successfully firing gate, lower the probability of change. (You can wangle this with changing your rules on your random number system.) At the non-excited gate, raise the probability of change. (The computer will tell us by how much eventually.) Raise sufficiency of all excited gates, make them more fussy. At mutual connections, let them go inhibitory, or raise their probability of turning inhibitory. All this to cells which fire only.

We now go on with the game and some other event comes up and is treated in a similar way. Eventually this first event comes again.

All the gates have got more fussy and they are tending to 'squash' one another's firing. The one that had the best initial fit has the best chance of surviving the battle for this particular event. Eventually, one of the gates will 'drop out' and not fire. If we get our rules right, the struggle for that event may go on for a time, but eventually one gate will have 'captured' it and, since it is constantly trying out variations of its unsuccessful inputs by raising the probability of change at them and lowering probability at successful ones, it will tend to get a better and better and fussier and fussier selector of the particular event. Now comes the tricky bit. Somehow or other it has got to stop raising sufficiency, getting fussy, or it will lose the event again. It has to stop it at a very precise point, at the point when it gets all or very nearly all the members of the 'class' within some tolerance. In the drawing, the class has only one member, but in real life there will be vague class boundaries and many slightly different input configurations will be proper (useful) members of the class. The correct adjustment of the sufficiency gate is a tricky matter and it will certainly never be a complete 'and' gate. I have no idea, at the moment of writing, how we can get over this, but we shall ask the computer if it can try out more different programs and metaprograms than I could in a lifetime. The basic idea is that in the unsophisticated visual cortex there is a set of transforms (changes of program) which will cause gates, call them neurons, to 'capture' a pattern if it is repeated often enough. My drawing is one-dimensional but it illustrates a two-dimensional array. Perceptual elements like 'short straight line' and 'black line termination' and so on can be discriminated and we have now created the first stratum.

Now look at the axonal end of this component. We need a different strategy. We need two kinds of input signals here, success and failure, pain and pleasure. Since we want the percept to grow towards the coincident motorium firing pattern, if it is successful, and to search elsewhere if it is a failure *i.e.* if the coincidental motor pattern *happens* to be wrong. We need some rule like: on success, distal facilitation, lateral inhibition; on failure, distal inhibition, lateral excitation. What this means simply is 'yes that works probe towards the motorium and try and make contact with whatever was going on when this successful thing happened', as when the baby got the nice taste from the chocolate drop. But when baby got a smack or the thing was not a chocolate drop but a razor blade, certainly it wants to know all about razor blades but the 'reaching for' behaviour idea is not a goer, so we cut off the probing towards the motorium and start a search laterally for a better coincident motor pattern next time.

This simple component can also be built up for a long sensorium, not as I have shown, with all gates looking at one set of neurons, but with a good deal of overlap. If systems such as I have shown were looking at the next group B,C,D,E,F,G,H,I, and another lot was looking at C,D,E,F,G,H,I,J, and so on, we have a rough bread-board model of what would produce the first stratum of the kind of polyhierarchic connectivity pattern I posit.

If, at a succession of strata, the outstretched dendrites, of more components collect together the axonal end connections, layer after layer, we will have, as the system adjusts, a similar pattern-grabbing competition; at the first stage for various assemblies of the first stratum axons, at the third of the second stratum axons and so on. The successive assembly of more and more repetitive pattern elements and assemblies proceeds by stages thus.

I predict that we shall find that there is such a set of rules which will create a polyhierarchic recognition system out of this approach. I cannot rule out that this has already been invented but I arrived at this idea from my meditations and from nowhere else. Popper may or may not feel that something will have been proved if my crude model neuron works. It is a rather elaborate 'failure to falsify', but a universe of evidence is the universe I happen to be living in, and I extend a very hearty welcome to Karl to come and join us all.

The answer to the wretched 'white swan' controversy that obsessed the *Philosophy of Science Journal* for many years is on similar lines. The argument goes thus, if I remember it rightly: the statement that, 'all swans are white', is logically equivalent to the statement that all non-white objects are non-swans. Then, we find a black shoe and say: Is this a confirmation of the hypothesis because it is a non-swan? And believe me, or believe me not, my beloved reader, paper after paper on this was published in the columns of that learned journal for years until I grew impatient of reading it. The answer is so simple. Yes, sure, it confirms it; but it does so to such an infinitesimal extent that it is not worth the ink in one full stop of one of the scores of papers on the subject, to say so. In the real universe, probabilities as low as that are meaningless. The procedure for confirming the hypothesis proposed is to look at every non-white item in the universe to check it. I would favour the strategy of inspecting swans. Lesson: if you really want to know something practical about the universe inspect the smallest, *i.e.*, least probable set which can tell you anything. I dare say I shall be drummed out of the Philosophy of Science Society now, but as the only member without an 'O' level, let alone a doctorate, I feel a bit of an intruder anyway. The whole thing is a terrible warning about mechanomorphic or determinist thinking. But after that diversion to reduce the tedium, let me return to my onions.

There is a difficulty which I have not cleared up and don't know how to ask the computer to clear up. The type of component I have described, my model neuron, has to go 'and-y' to get fussy and discriminitive or, 'or-y' and become a 'generalization' gate. Now generalization is enormously economical from the point of view of information theory. An 'or'-type generalization centre can bring together connections from all the loci where the concepts 'spoon' may occur and link that with the motor pattern 'saying spoon', the auditory locus 'sound of the word spoon' and tactile locus 'feel of a spoon' at an even more general gate 'spoon'. At an even higher level 'and' gate the 'spoon' locus can be used recombinatively to create a higher level 'and' centre where 'the spoon in my cup at this table at this time in this context', can be activated. This is a 'whole' event for a human being.

The problem is that though it is fairly clear intuitively that generalization or 'or'-type gates have got to be central, or tend to be more numerous in central apical regions, there has to be some kind of definable rule, or possibly a different kind of gate, which tells some gates to specialize in or-ness or generalization and others to get more 'and-y', fussy and discriminatory. In the one case sufficiency rises with success and in the other, somehow, it has to fall. Multiplexing might help here. A generalization gate is really a 'zone of greatest mutual interconnectivity', which itself gradually gets more fussy in rejecting inappropriate connections but responding to any appropriate ones. I have not solved this. I do not know how to ask the computer to solve it. I invite computer experts to think about it.

In the usual way of looking at things we have only to find one 'fatal flaw' and the whole theory goes overboard, but by my way of looking at things we go on trying a little more to see if we can find some definable rules which would help us. All hypotheses, even successful ones, find themselves, in the end, *ad hoc*-ing around, as their imperfections appear. Eventually the whole thing gets ridiculous, as with the Ptolomaic astronomic model and we have to have a new one because we cannot go on patching the old one any longer. In comes Copernicus and we find a better approximation which goes very well till we find some untidy bits and need Kepler. Later, remaining oddities in the bit of the Keplerian model with the real world make a new model, that of Einstein necessary, and so on.

At any rate, generalization reduces the complexity of the problem, the variety of inputs and the probability of successful recognition.

What we are doing as we go up the strata is filtering out our doubts. The higher we go, the greater the specification and the more tolerance or lower sufficiency we can get on with without raised probability of error. The brain is an uncertainty valve or filter letting in only useful, valid and predictive (because repetitive) information and filtering out noise, irrelevant, superfluous, information. We start with the instrument, a receptor, looking at a spot which is some shade of grey and saying, 'is this black or white?'. We finish with one decision: 'Order Fifth Battalion to Advance', and the *gestalters* tell me that it is all done at one stage!

The central problem, unsolved, is what is the difference in rule which gets us two opposite trends: (a) generalization 'or'-type connections and, (b) recombination assemblies of generalizations, like language, like phrases such as 'small bent silver spoon on the window sill'; a new kind of highly specified class made up of an assembly of generalizations. Problem unsolved: over to you. But am I asking a productive question?

Another problem: I have taken the success/failure signals a bit for granted up to now. One thing we know for sure is that there is a rack-renting system in acquiring skills; a 'get more fussy' system. Performances which we consider successful when we first start learning, disgust us after more learning. So there must be a raising of the threshold of 'expectation' whatever that may mean. If these hierarchies grow from the base too, this is consonant with what goes before. Somewhere there is a success and failure threshold setting system which, like a sufficiency gate, raises targets systematically on success. I had thought about this as a ubiquitous signal probably applying everywhere, another input to every connection of every gate. It may be a chemical condition in surrounding glial cells? This could have a differential effect according to whether or not the cell had recently fired and whether the programme was positive or negative at the synapse. The 'pleasure' and 'pain' centres which have been found in the brain are helpful here but how do they send their message to every synapse quickly enough? What is quickly enough? How long does it take to 'learn' (as distinct from 'make a new connection')? My guess is about half an hour and this means that the programme box or synapse has to 'remember' conditions for about that time.

But this 'rack-renting' is a visible aspect in well-managed firms. Accountants ask for 'projections'. Each department sets itself targets as optimistic as possible. The manager goes for his target and, if he reaches it, is given a pat on the back, a rise and a new, higher target. The man who is too optimistic falls short, gets a mild or severe rebuke but may talk his way into a slightly lower, more realistic target. Orgs are orgs. These are not analogies. We are talking about widely different members of a valid natural class of entity. A class of morphostats trying to be better ones.

Prediction

Penfield says that, at least in the speech areas, cortical stimulation cannot elicit the performance of elementary sub-skills such as the pronouncing of a word or phrase (but vocalization *can* be produced). I predict that, perhaps in insects at first, activation centres will be found which, by being stimulated, will trigger complex behaviour patterns.

One demonstration that the recognition process must be analytical comes from the rapidly developing science of pattern or, to avoid argument, figure recognition. (A figure is a pattern with semantic content). Development of this art is disappointingly slow. At this stage the probability of error in wide tolerance recognition is still too high for practical purposes, but the successful approach has been that of searching the field for the presence of perceptual elements and then checking whether there are sufficient and whether they have the right orientation.

A rueful story told by those in the field is that an elaborate pattern recognition circuit was set up. It had as its receptor a television camera. Due to the uncertainty of its response the connected computer was empowered to give its answers with varying degrees of certainty. It could say 'this is probably an x', 'this might be an x', and so on. The great day came and the camera was presented with a tennis ball as the object it had to recognize. For half an hour the computer worked impassively rotating its tape wheels and blinking its lights in taciturn activity. Then the printout typewriter began to rattle 'This *might* be an egg'. However the recognition of typewritten letters has now reached the point where the probability of error is as low as 20 negabits or a million to one against. And it has been done by a 3 stratum machine with tolerance at each stratum which is looking for 'features'. The work of Dr Parks of the British National Physical Laboratory shows this. In character recognition, features such as mid cross ('+'), upper termination, lower termination, 'dark high horizontal edge', are sought electronically and used to recognize alphanumeric characters.

Postscript, April 1975

My speculations have led to results more tangible than this book. They have also led to a feasibility study by Howell and Matthews of Plesseys which is now complete.

They have developed electronic 'hardware' which can compete successfully with the human timber-grader in recognizing, measuring, and locating defects in softwood. Live and dead knots, rot, sapstain, cross-grain, wane, and splits can be distinguished, measured and located at 3m/sec.

A field trial machine will be complete before next year.

Chapter 10 Implications

Having unburdened myself, in an undisciplined way, I am afraid, of the essentials of an idea, I want to follow some of its implications for those who feel it may have some merit. The implications are considerable. To me they seem to throw a different light on many things.

Since I have been talking about the hardware or the physical components which may demonstrate the validity of my simple basic hypothesis let me look now at the possibilities that arise in the field of computers.

Towards an Electronic Brain

Traditional computers can be made to simulate some of the functions of the brain but there is little similarity. The computer is a finite-state machine. The number of ways in which its components can be arranged is large but not without limit. Brains, the biological and sociological type, are, for all practical purposes, infinite-state machines. Even if the component, the neuron, has only two states, more variety creeps in because the rates of firing are variable. The number of components is so large that, even without variable firing rates, the distinction between the number of possible states of the system and infinity could not possibly be of human significance. A traditional computer is essentially monolinear. It has a single, or very few, inputs that operate simultaneously, whereas the brain has a vast number of parallel inputs. A computer is determinist. It apes the strictly causal universe which is assumed by scientists to be the real one, but which Heisenberg has shown is not. A brain is stochastic. It is an odds-estimating machine as Gray Walter has said, like a 'row of bookmakers'. A computer is good at chain thinking, logical processes, deduction. The brain works on inference and evidence, balancing credibilities and probabilities. A computer uses trigger action to eliminate random noise. Pulses are squared and tidied up at each regeneration. The brain uses random noise and amplifies it to create curiosity, exploration and experiment. It is an array of Maxwell demons, using information to create and contain order and its atomic equivalent, energy. But it is not because computers are machines that they are as they are, it is because we built them to solve the problems that we find most difficult, logical, deductive, mathematical ones. The input of the traditional computer is encoded predigested data. Computers cannot solve the interface problem. But, as pattern recognition develops we shall have computers with many simultaneous input and output connections: computers which can work direct from raw data, meter readings, point intensities. Computers which can formulate and test hypotheses, balance odds and optimize decisions. And carry them out.

And this, as I. J. Good has said is the first step in an Intelligence Explosion. Man designs stochastic computers. These design better ones and these, better ones still. The first steps of a terrifying infinite regression. Will Man become redundant? We had better watch that he does not. There is no immediate worry. A cost/benefit exercise will quickly show that the old-fashioned way of reproducing brains is still cheapest as well as the more enjoyable.

But the one thing we can get from electronic brains is impartiality. In government and management today we find it hard to get brains to work to agreed goals without distortions due to self interest. The selfishness of all élites is the basic problem of politics. But you cannot corrupt a computer and we trust them accordingly. We sit at a traffic light for instance, quietly obedient to its often rather silly instructions. If a policeman held us up for nothing to pass we should report him.

The Implications for Politics
Conservatism and Conservation.

The acceptance of these views involves sociological conclusions which are extremely unpalatable in this age. But I have been justifying something that was taken for granted by most people in most ages. The stability-seeking aspect of human groups and societies has always been the most evident aspect. There has never been an age when the innate conservatism of living groups of men has been less that it is now. As far back into the past as we can see, men living in families, tribes, groups, villages, towns, have been obsessively and rigidly conservative. The hard-won heredity of knowledge, skills, habits and behaviour patterns which had brought a group safely through, against all the odds, to whatever point in time or whatever state of organization it had reached, was prized above all else. The young men listened to the elders and the elders were guided by religions, rites, rituals, precedents tales, stories, and a thousand dramatic tricks to preserve viable behaviour patterns. Much of the resultant behaviour was ritualistic nonsense, unnecessary. But no one knew the contingent from the necessary and all was retained. Sir Arthur Keith tells us of the way people lived before the great changes started, with the development of agriculture, 6 or 7 kiloyear ago. Here and there in the world, even today, there are pockets of humanity living in the same ancient way; cut-off tribes in Africa and New Guinea and in the deep forests of the Amazon. Margaret Mead, Malinowsky and other anthropologists have studied these societies closely and though many will doubt that a tribe under study is the same thing as a tribe period, the overall scheme is clear. It is similar to that uncovered by the zoologists and the newer breed, ethologists, who are investigating the behaviour of the animals in the wild.

The living space is divided into a network of well-defined tribal areas.

Each tribe lives in a state of variable but more or less constant enmity with its neighbours, it repels them and is repelled by them. The means of repulsion is largely ritualistic fighting. What traffic the neighbouring tribes have is conducted in an atmosphere of rigid ritual and formality and seems to be concerned with an outbreeding pattern necessary to preserve the gene pools from faults which develop if they become too small.

The life of the 'noble savage' was not what the encyclopaedists and modern anarchists suppose. Their life was not solitary, nor brutish, but it is poor, nasty and short. They suffer from many ills and scratch a poor and uncertain living from gathering and hunting. They are haunted by ghosts and taboos. Their life is governed by the rigid behaviour patterns they have inherited. Take a tribesman away from his own area into the no-mans-land between the tribal areas and his fear grows until it is insupportable and he flees back to his own country. But the whole network is in fact a symbiotic self-adjusting system and the pattern of tribes is in stable long-term ecological balance with the terrain, its fauna and flora. While the sun shines on the earth the pattern could continue indefinitely. The fear of strangers and of the unfamiliar together with the uncomprehended mechanisms of social heredity, custom, taboo and religion, have created a self organizing pattern of life which, though none too pleasant, must be accorded a respectability based on the length of time for which it has successfully survived. Mankind has survived a succession of civilizations but we cannot point to any civilization which has defied time to any real extent. Certainly, by all the auguries, the latest flowering of the interaction and communication of men, our present world civilization, has no promise of permanence or stability.

The neglected Keith and the rejected Darlington point out that it is from this pattern that all past civilizations have emerged. It is also clear that it is for this pattern that the animal Man is most suited. All civilizations have proved to be ephemeral and after all but the last man has reverted to the territorial pattern. But, since the development of agriculture, there have been accumulations of cultural information which have provided an advanced new starting point for each next adventure into the use of third-order intelligence. The primitive pattern, where lives were poor, nasty and short for men and women, made lives which were long, stable and viable for super-orgs, the groupings in which they lived.

The territorial, hunter-gatherer tribes are, relative to our new-fangled nations, immortal; of their eventual survival we are surest.

I am looking upon the individual as the substrate or pabulum upon which such orgs as cultures, tribes, societies grow, and seeing the cultural organization supported by tribal mores, or patterns of communication, as third-order orgs growing in a medium of human beings. These super-orgs are evolving, breeding, living and dying. So the primitive, pre-protoplasmic matter may have behaved when the first life forms were emerging.

Each sociological experiment emerges from the one before, has its babyhood, youth, manhood, senility and death.

From this point of view, the occasional brief, unstable, upflare of a human civilization might be looked at as a predator to which the normal third-order pattern is prone. A growing together and proliferation which is as yet unstable: the whole thing an unfortunate side effect of the large and efficient brain which even the primitive tribal man had to evolve to survive in the competitive, adventurous, non-specialist, niche-transcending niche among animals which he has occupied. What are we to say about the latest example of this infection, today's world civilization. A giant super-org has enveloped the globe, a runaway growth, a cancer?

There can be no profit in accepting such a dismal conclusion. This ugly idea is based upon observation of the past and trends which are manifest. But, with living systems, it is just the observation that a thing will probably happen which prevents its happening. Information moves into the polyhierarchic system and the org lurches into a counteracting modality. If the rapid increase in exchange of information that is going on in the world-wide link-up of the minds of men constitutes a primitive brain of a fourth-order org then, against all probability, it will, as every living thing does from moment to moment in time, win the long-odds battle against the great weight of statistical probability. Like every living thing we shall, whether we want to or not, fight to the last gasp to preserve the form of our great civilization.

The Implications for Organization Theory

What is an organization? It is the name of a class with high tolerance, wide boundaries. It includes everything from the oldest organization, probably the Catholic Church, to the group of strangers which gathers round a traffic accident to help. An organization is an assembly of co-operating people. In the original form of organization there was but one primary purpose, survival. To achieve survival, not merely the group of individuals; but the patterns of cooperation between them; have to be preserved. The codes, mores, religions, morals – they have many names – have to be conserved with minimum change because the more viable a thing is, the more likely it is that a change will make it less viable. Like other orgs, an organization must preserve its form through time and accept only those changes which make it a better form-preserving device. As I have said, organizations must be and are conservative. But, as we have seen with more complex but lower-level orgs such as cells and animals, the most rigid system is not always the most viable. Organizations, like other orgs, must have a means of generating randomness, experimental changes, and selecting from them. They must accept only those modifications which improve change-resisting ability. To do this they have the same problem as any other org; they have to receive, classify, evaluate and condense incoming information and transduce it into appropriate instructions to members. The problem of separating organizations conceptually from their environment, the even larger org, society, is difficult.

Within them there is a specially rich flow of information but they themselves are deeply embedded in and closely entwined as regards the flow of information with the larger organizations of which they form part. The information that passes into them and out of them is true information. It is encoded. It is not signals coming from meter readings, point-intensities in the world. Much of the instruction which flows out from them in coded form does not trigger motor action until it has passed through one or more links in other organizations.

The reader will remember looking at an animal and being asked to perform upon it a messy topological operation. First I rolled it up into a ball with a spotted surface. Then I peeled away the muscles and receptors until I had nothing but nerve endings, afferent and efferent on the surface of a sphere. Then I patted the sphere into a cube and pulled all the afferent nerve endings to one surface and the efferent nerve endings to the opposite one. I did not change the connections but the operation was a major one, drastic conceptual surgery! To perform this operation with an organization is much less simple. Firstly, its junction point – its cells – are people, each with their own elaborate

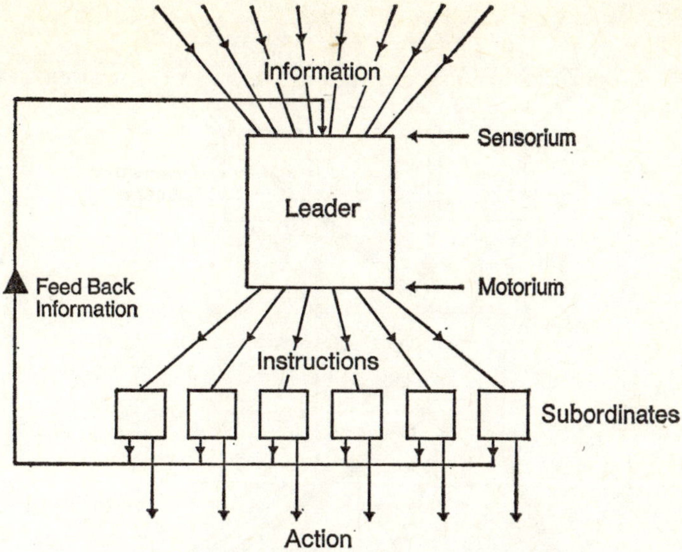

Fig. 26a The growth of an organization, stage 1

sensorium and motorium; and secondly, the placental connections with the rest of society at the sensorium of the organization and at its motorium are more difficult to disentangle. In Fig. 26 we can see the first three stages of the growth of an organization.

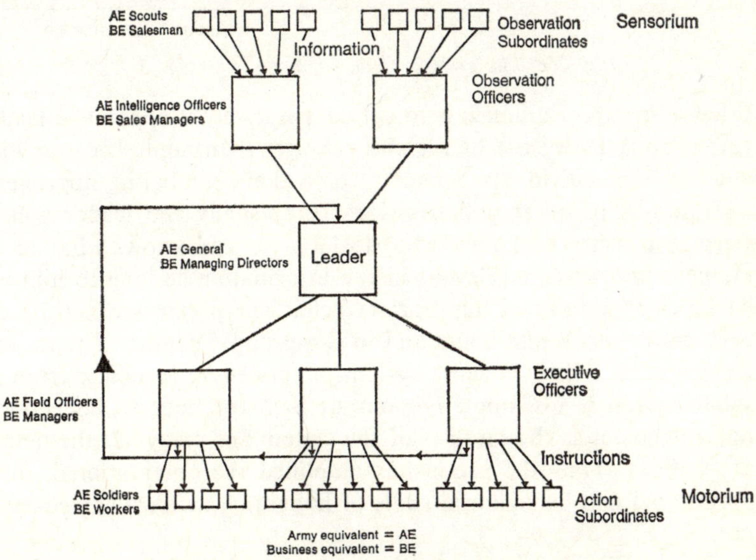

Fig. 26b The growth of an organization, stage 2

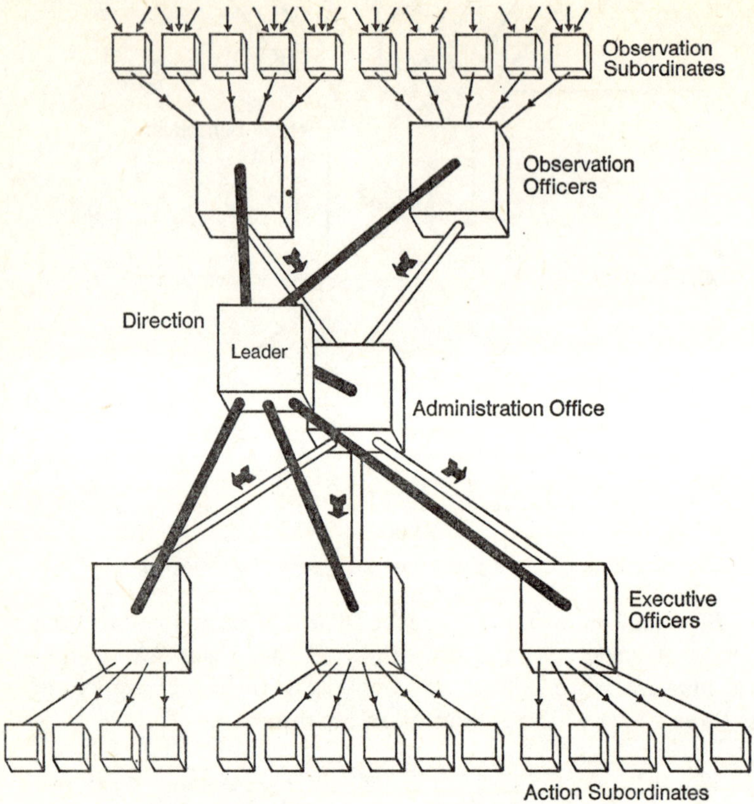

Fig. 26c The growth of an organization, stage 3

When a group of animals is to act cooperatively it appoints a leader, patent or tacit. Even a bad leader is better than none, because without one the individuals cannot resolve their conflicting approaches with sufficient speed and decision. But usually the leader will be selected because he knows what to look for and knows what to do. He perceives what is relevant in the information coming to him and he has a repertoire of appropriate behaviour patterns which he can perform or teach and command in the group. Diagram 1 represents the situation. His own sense system, amplified by feedback from his subordinates, is his input. His output is instructions to his subordinates, who act as the muscles of the system and carry out the necessary actions. Thus the group has amplified the observational, interpretational and behavioural skills of hopefully, its most skilled member.

In Stage 2, Fig. 26b organization has become larger as the number of people the leader has to deal with has become too great. He is now unable to cope with the flow of information. He appoints agents on both sides of himself; afferent and efferent. The observation officers select and condense the incoming information, predigesting it to diminish his information load.

On the efferent side, an elaborative hierarchy expands, amplifies and develops his instructions and passes them to last line subordinates, who carry them out.

The same features arise in any kind of organization, but they are often named in different ways. The Army and business equivalents, for various roles are given.

In the third stage, Fig. 26c organization has grown still further and despite the arrangements in stage 2, the leader is overloaded once more, from an information point of view. He can no longer deal even with the refined and condensed convergent information and he can no longer issue even those key instructions which require a further elaboration.

He develops an administrative office with a number of subordinates who carry out the routine aspects of his responsibilities. Now only low probability, non-routine matters are referred to him. At later stages, many specialized hierarchies develop, which overlie the principal authority hierarchy. For instance, in the British Army structure, the specialist corps (Signals, Education, Intelligence) represent multiple, separate hierarchies.

A commercial firm, is something that can clearly be seen to be unitary despite the complexity of its informational connections. The reason we have no difficulty in separating it conceptually is because it has a relatively independent array of decision centres, and acts principally and mainly in its own interests and in the direction of its own survival. Ostensibly, it will have other aims connected with its function in the society to which it belongs but its 'will to live' is almost always much more important than any of its members see. Organizations continue to exist long after the need for them has vanished and others exist like an animal for no reason at all except that they can. Donald Schon, in his Reith Lectures, pointed out that many organizations reach their most mature form and most elaborate development long after the reasons for which they were set up have vanished. The ostensible aims are often very different from the true ones. The local office of a political party, except at election time, is a social bickering club for the discharge of now useless aggression. As Darlington points out, religions exist ostensibly to pay tribute to phantom projections of man in the heavens, but their true role is the same as the nucleus of the cell, organization and cohesion, the passing on of an inheritance of information patterns and a sense of who is 'us' and who is 'them' which seems essential to human cooperation; a pattern clearly linked to the territorial, mutually repelling groups. At the biological level the organism as a whole must provide sustenance for its cells, which have specialized and lost the power of independent life. Morphostats must be viable at all levels.

Similarly, in organizations, the individual must gain from his cooperation. He must be provided with sustenance or satisfaction to retain his adhesion. I have defined a need as a threat to the stability of an org. The elements of an org, as well as the org itself, have needs. The needs are not necessarily the same. Indeed, they are often contradictory. Human beings have not only needs but aspirations and, in this context, an aspiration is a need for progress, security, a move towards a more stable configuration. When the primary needs of members of organizations are satisfied, then one aspiration, that for greater security, asserts itself.

Orgs as primitive and as loosely coupled as human organizations suffer from a difficulty which is not, because of long evolution and compromise adaption, so evident in more developed but lower level orgs. The needs and aspiration of members of organizations are *often* not compatible and even contradict the needs of the organization as a whole. The primary problem of an organizer is that of achieving the optimum compromise satisfaction of the needs and aspirations of role incumbents at all levels, which is compatible with the stability, continuation and progress of the organization itself. A glance at the diseases of organizations, the faulty patterns which bring them to an end at either extreme will demonstrate the point. Where the managers of any organization err on the side of paying too much attention to the individual's needs and aspirations, the organization ceases to be viable. Even if it does survive, it is directionless and impotent.

At the other extreme, organizations, in emergency or under attack, become more sensitive to central signals. Individual needs and aspirations are reduced, discipline becomes severe; loss and sacrifice are accepted by individuals for the benefit of the group. An army at war is an example. To achieve this predominance of central control; centreproneness, there is in mankind, says Lorenz, a different modality, a behaviour pattern which is switched on in certain circumstances; the Military Enthusiasm of which Lorenz writes. Even so, there is an extreme of centre-proneness which will destroy an organization. Discipline which is too strict leads to repression and punishment. The proprioceptive feedback signals are over-inhibited and revolt, mutiny or revolution eventually results. But we seem to have forgotten, in this age, the incredible altruism which extreme discipline can produce without breakdown. It depends on the urgency of the threat. C. S. Forester's 'Hornblower' series reminds us how strong can be the discipline a group can viably survive.

Organs

The word organization comes from the word organ and the word can be used in the sense 'form organs'. An organ is that part of an entity which specializes in dealing with certain types of problem, certain types of threat of change. The nucleus, the brain of a cell, contains the instructions which enable it to form the specialist parts required to deal with the threats that will probably exist in its particular environment. A system of chromosomes is, in a very real sense, 'aware' of the environment in which the org will live. It would be possible to 'deduce' the environment by a sufficiently informed examination of the genetic code material. In the organization, aside from the knowledge stored in the brains of the individual members, there is immanent in the pattern of organization an understanding of the social environment in which the organization works. The type of organizational centres, the pattern and flow of information, the connections and deconnections, result from the interaction of a large number of people over a period of time. This is an inductive 'learning' process. Organizations 'learn' at an unconscious meta-level. A recursive, self-correcting system modifies the network in ways which are by no means apparent to those who suppose themselves to be in command. Each individual receives and deals with information and passes it on according to what he has been taught and the necessities of the moment. The flow of information to him grows and shrinks and he reacts to this. Unexpected links and bypasses spring up. Information moves in unorthodox directions. The flow of information is often not directed by any one person's decision, but by the necessities of the situation and a multiplicity of decisions in many places. In this sense organizations, especially large ones, are self-organizing systems, orgs, morphostats.

Traditional View of Organization as Monohierarchic

The traditional view of organization was first clarified in Roman times.

The basic concept is that of responsibility. The question asked is: 'who is compelled to supply answers to whom?' The role of questioner is the role of mastery. The answerer's role is one of subjection. In any entity which has the problem of amplifying uncertainty so as to build improbable arrangements, the first problem is to build an amplification system. Systems in which all elements are equivalent are not and cannot be organized. We can have societies in which all men's rights are equal but we cannot have an *organization* in which the effect of all men is equal. We can have organizations in which every member has a voice in deciding who will be the leaders. We cannot have organizations, viable ones, of any size at any rate, without leadership. Leadership is a device invented, unconsciously, to provide the necessary trigger effect, the necessary amplification, the necessary non-equivalence of the elements of any morphostatic system. A leader is a decision gate, a trigger or relay. So is a committee. The gate receives information from many sources, makes a decision and transmits information transduced into negative and positive instructions. The similarity between the leader and the central decision gates I have postulated in the polyhierarchic network is obvious. But, at first sight, he seems to be the apex of a single hierarchy. We shall see.

Development from Monohierarchic to Polyhierarchic organization

It goes without saying that the random behaviour of a mob is different in a very profound sense from the behaviour of a body of organized men. Leadership is an ubiquitous feature of any body of organized men of any size or complexity. It has been argued that gangs or teams do exist and function without visible leadership, that small, face-to-face groups can work cooperatively in pre-allocated roles without visible leadership, but on a large scale, the pattern is rare and its converse almost universal.

The problem of any leader is that of changing the behaviour of his followers from what it would have been without him, towards conformity with one of a repertoire of highly-specified combined patterns of corporate behaviour. The leader acts as a decision gate. He defines and allocates roles, (functions). He receives evidence from his own sensorium and this is supplemented by pre-coded information coming from some of his followers. He makes his decision on the balance of the evidence and then issues a different kind of information, *instructions* of an appropriate kind to the followers. The followers conform to assigned roles. They are both receptors and effectors. But the leader himself has a brain and within it are stored a set of sets of instructions each suitable for a different decision. If he is the captain of a ship he has a repertoire of 'whole situation' navigating behaviour patterns. He has the set of orders he would give for 'heave to', the set of orders for 'set sail', the set of orders to deal with a storm, the set of orders to deal with fog, and so on. He does not know and need not know all the detailed actions involved in the carrying out of his orders. The instructions are simple but the activities they evoke are complex in terms of the instructions eventually sent to the muscles of the sailor. The apparently monohierarchic system is polyhierarchic at least at the centre. As soon as the organization grows beyond a certain point the flow of information through the leader gets to be more than he can handle and he begins to delegate. He delegates both on the afferent and the efferent side of himself, though the same person may act in two different roles, the role of information-giver and the role of instruction-collector.

The examination of any large organization will reveal that as it gets larger it gets more polyhierarchic, more and more offices and centres form on which information on certain matters and subdivisions of work converge and from which instructions are issued automatically under the general authority of the management but without information passing through the managerial part of the channel.

The *good* manager is a supervisor of the *network*, not of the contents, the information. He does not insert himself into the flow of information. One of the serious faults of an organization is that which develops when a manager fails to arrange adequate bypasses to himself and insists on trying to channel all information through himself and issue all instructions from himself. He is sticking to the method of the primitive face-to-face group and it is unsuitable when the information flow, both afferent and efferent, is at more than a certain level.

Large monohierarchic organizations have proved to be unstable and relatively inefficient. The strictly monohierarchic organization of the Aztec and Inca civilizations, although they were very elaborate and highly structured, collapsed ignominiously at the first contact with a Western polyhierarchy.

The Roman pattern of organization was a development from the primitive one-to-many-flow-of-instruction pattern. It was an amplification system. The hierarchical structure arose when the initial array of instruction receivers began to develop their own subordinates and radiate the instructions wider and wider. It was this pattern that made it possible for mankind to live symbiotically in large groups. It was this epoch-making discovery that created third-order orgs which grew upon the substrate of primitive tribal society.

But the same pattern can be seen in the offices of every company. Look at the familiar hierarchic organization chart. It represents the *authority* structure. It is a picture of both afferent and efferent sides of the communications network mixed up. It leads down to the motorium and sensorium combined in one line. It takes no account of the sensorium in its external divergence out beyond the 'Sales Department'. In these charts, the 'Sales' side and the 'Works' side, the apical sensory regions and the apical motor regions, are shown as part of the same hierarchy despite the fact that, broadly speaking, the flow of information is afferent in one case and efferent in the other.

The normal organization chart usually shows a long box at the top called, 'the shareholders' or the 'electorate', as the source of the central authority exerted by the 'President' or 'Managing Director' or whoever occupies the single role box below it. Those acquainted with the functioning of large companies will know that the effect of signals from the central authority 'shareholders' or 'electorate' on the day-to-day or even the year-to-year functioning of the organization is negligible; except in dire failure situations, when the death of the org is near. Signals converging from electorates and shareholders are so rare, so unorganized, so confused and so crude that they do not have a significant influence on the decision makers. It is only when *organizations* like lobbies, pressure groups, trade unions and similar associations with their own hierarchic structures grow up that their signals begin to impinge with any force on the central decision making processes. The traditional model of organization is incomplete because it partly leaves out the afferent side and muddles it with the efferent side, and it is inaccurate because the flow of information and instruction is just not like that. The traditional picture of the boss who is supposed to have a one-way influence on the behaviour of those in the stratum below him and of those in the next stratum, in their turn controlling behaviour of the stratum below, is based on an earlier pattern where it was possible for the man at the top to observe and remember everything so that he needed no information collecting hierarchies.

The development of the polyhierarchic pattern began when the persons in the second stratum were appointed. Because of special skills and abilities which the top man did not fully understand, they bypass the boss and give orders directly. The second stratum experts had to have information and they began to develop their own information-collecting hierarchies. These are also a bypass to the top man. The subordinate is not now acting only under signals from the top but he is receiving other afferent information which bypasses and may be incomprehensible to the man at the top. This is illustrated in Fig. 26c. With elaboration, this then develops to the situation in Fig. 27 as the subordinates' input hierarchy grows.

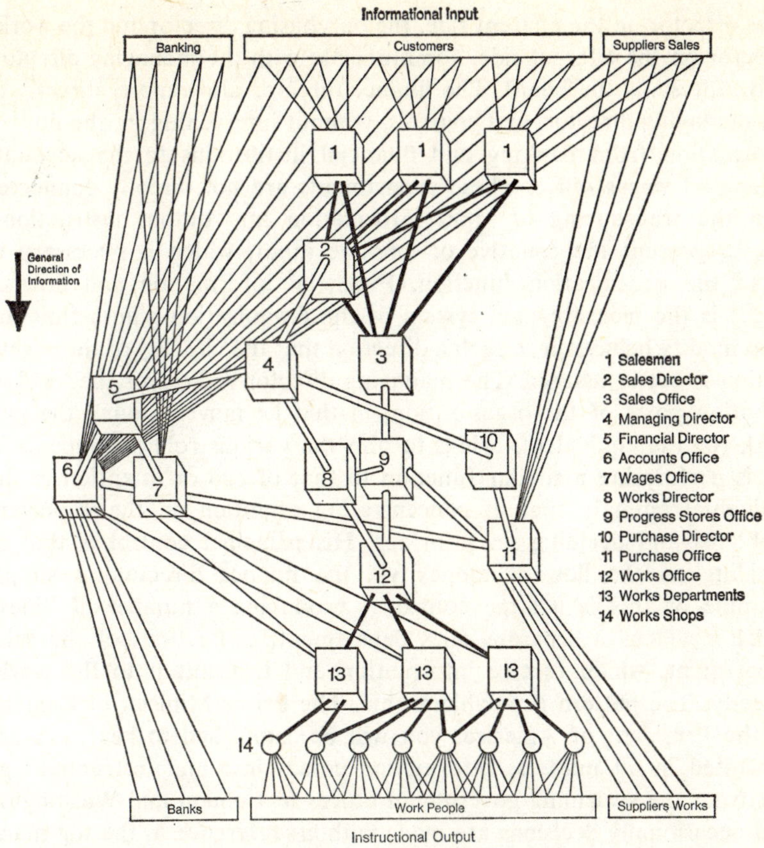

Fig. 27 Informational structure of a typical manufacturer. The main flow of information/instruction is in the lowest plane. Top management structure is best seen as an overpass system. Only principal channels are shown. All are two-way, but general direction is from sensorium to motorium.

In Fig. 27 I have tried to show where some of the officers in a small manufacturing company fit into the polyhierarchic informational structure which I propose. The informational input comes from banking and financial institutions, customers and the sales departments of suppliers. The total input converges on sales offices, purchasing offices and accounts and wages departments. The principal information from the sales office passes to the progress office, stores, etc, departments where the work is planned. From there it goes to the works office, is issued to works departments and at a lower strata, to workshops and finally to the workpeople. Other information from progress office goes to the purchasing office, from which instructions are issued to the works supplying company. The three principal operational directors – the sales director on the afferent side, the purchasing director and the works director on the efferent side, communicate with the managing director, who represents the board. The finance director also reports directly to the managing director, and controls, without intervening in, the flow of information from banking and financial institutions to the accounts office and wages office. These departments are not directly connected with the transducing of input information into output instructions. They represent the conative or emotive input, which is necessary to make the organization function. Financial information and flow of wages is the pleasure/pain system of the organization whose function is to modify behaviour in such a direction that the viability of the organization is better assured. The managing director represents the 'ego' or attention point of the organization, in that he moves around the network (or the equivalent, brings to him the various role incumbents in it), is performing a similar function to that of ego or attention in the individual animal: that of concentrating attention on the important problems and deciding on priorities. His principal control is that of deciding on the flow of money via the finance director. A simple example of this is a large company, producing a number of 'lines', which develops a separate sales department, or sections of the sales department, which receive information and transmit it to the works directly. The pattern is polyhierarchic. The Prime Minister of England or the President of America, you will be astonished to hear, are not consulted in all matters. Information comes into and instructions go out from the swarming government offices in London and Washington and occasionally decisions are made without reference to the top man!

What, then, is the role of the 'top man' in the large organization? We know of very few examples of viable organizations which do not have an extremely obvious 'top man'. Why? The value of the top man to the organization may be partly as a focus of loyalty. Must there be an incumbent of the 'old man' role because it is traditional and psychologically necessary for the majority of the members of the organization whose understanding is anthropomorphic?

There is a much more functional need for a boss. Let us trace the development. As the organization grows, a point is reached in which the boss becomes a decision bottleneck. He simply has not enough time to absorb all the information and issue all the instructions needed. Since he, at this stage is the repository of the essential data, he develops hierarchies on both the afferent and the efferent side of himself. Specialist information collectors, specialist instruction issuers. Eventually he is repeatedly bypassed and the organization reaches an autonomic stage. The central management is then pushed by the necessities of the information flow situation to one of a number of different roles. Another aspect of the boss's function begins to be paramount. It is the supervision of the reward and punishment system. Animals have pain and pleasure, organizations have to have their parallel reward and punishment systems to reinforce appropriate, successful behaviour and inhibit inappropriate, unsuccessful behaviour. I do *so* apologize for this unfashionable view. But the manager has to convert the random self-regarding behaviour patterns of a large number of people into the highly specified behaviour patterns required by the organization. Really.

The role of top management, when a company or organization reaches the autonomic stage, is more that of the success measuring, and the reward punishment system. The word punishment is unrespectable today, but it undoubtedly still occurs in all organizations. Those whose behaviour patterns do not conform to what is required are 'punished' in more subtle and evasive ways, but punished they are. Those whose efforts are notably successful are rewarded. Another role of the central management in large organizations is that of arousal and inhibition. The attention of the boss moves around among the internal decision centres, reshaping, rather than intervening in, the information flow. He directs the flow of excitatory and inhibitory instructions in this way: As he moves his attention from point to point in the network he is, in the light of some overall conception of policy, saying yes or no to elaborate preformed schemes. He is in effect the homologue of the attention point which I was discussing earlier. He is the excitatory augmentation which is required before certain kinds of non-routine activity can be undertaken. He is the long-term view man, the opportunity (and risk) taker. The final gate, trigger to *conscious* as distinct from autonomic or subconscious behaviour. He is the primitive beginning of a consciousness in the org.

Two Strata Hierarchies Inadequate

The concept of control directly from the base, as in a referendum, or via a two strata monohierarchic system via representatives as in democracy, will be seen from an informational point of view to fit very badly into the existing organizational structure of society. I say more of this later. The pressure of the citizens is certainly exerted, but it is influentially exerted by them in their role as consumers and by the way in which they spend their money, which passes up through a polyhierarchic structure, of retailers, wholesalers, to an apical region of manufacturers from which it cascades outwards until it reaches the same base or array of human beings from which it started in the form of instructions to them in their working roles. It is convenient and more

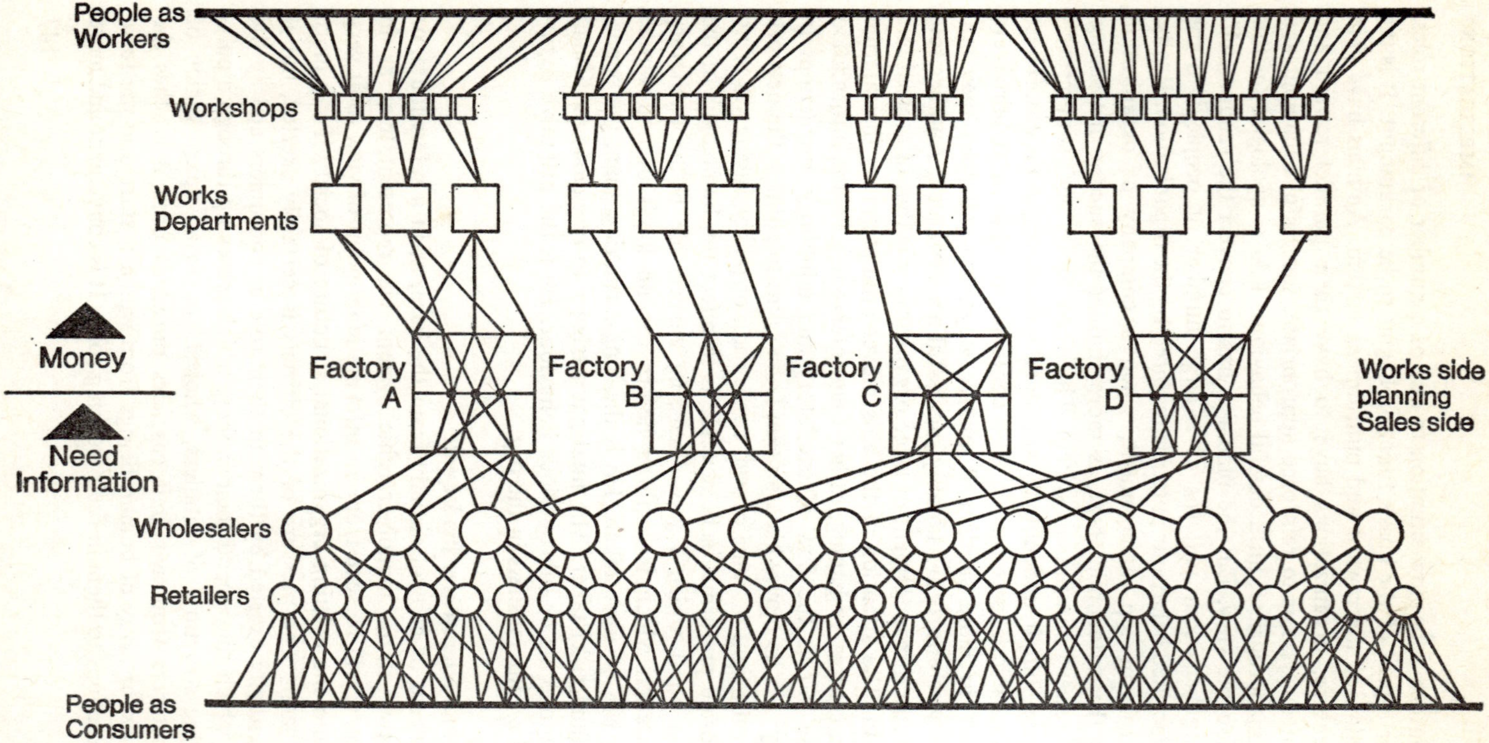

Fig. 28 Polyhierarchic flow of information in commercial transactions. 'Licensed need signals', money, flow from people in their consumer role, back to themselves as consumers.

predictive for us to separate the consumer role from the producer role in each person as in Fig. 28.

We are entitled to do this if it helps us to understand. It is visibly true that the behaviour patterns and the whole environment of each person in a modern society, has two aspects; he has two completely separate roles, the 'at-home-in-the-family, consumer', role and the 'at-work, producer' role. The conceptual separation is not an impermissible one. The picture given of the flow of information is broadly true and I believe it makes it much easier to grasp what is really happening in these highly complex systems. But every time we take nature apart to look at it, every time we insert our conceptual surgeon's knife to uncover the informational anatomy, we falsify, so there is a weakness in the simple polyhierarchic model which must be pointed out.

To make an organization's structure viable, the incumbent of every role at every level is, in fact, in two-way communication with those in the level below and above him. Proprioceptive feedback information is being sent back which affects the decisions which are made at a very local level. There are, for instance, afferent feedback signals from the muscle spindles of an animal which feed, directly to the motoneurons, local information about the state of extension of the muscle.

Similarly a workman may feed back to a foreman information which affects the foreman's decision on the spot. To fit this into the picture drawn we have to allow for bypass connections at all levels. The apices at quite low strata on the afferent side may have direct connections with apices at low strata on the efferent side. This does not invalidate the general picture. It is merely an extension of it.

A preferable way of looking at the matter might be the reverse. We might think of the primitive pattern of organization as this type of autonomic close, low-stratum connection. We could imagine a primitive organism or organization where the peripheral war with entropy consisted of a large number of local skirmishes with little central coordination. The development of the polyhierarchical structure I have proposed would be an outgrowth and development of this one-to-one autonomic system in which, as it were, each organ had its own receptor system. To make this point, I shall change the context.

Management

What more has my hypothesis got to say to the organization manager, to the boss, leader, dictator, prime minister?

Let us look a little more closely at the model of the brain. The linkages are at a succession of levels. The simple polyhierarchic picture was an oversimplification. A less simple oversimplification would be an evolution like this. First, simply a polycentric system, with various sensorium configurations connecting to motor-exciting centres at a central apical region. The next stage development is a 'flat' polyhierarchic network. A few strata with connections deterministic and action more or less 'reflex'. This system deals with events of high probability. But, as orgs learn to deal with events of lower and lower probability, they develop further polyhierarchic systems arching over one another and having a much larger number of apices. Another way of drawing it would be a polyhierarchic network growing upwards and outwards and proliferating apices, but with straight through-connections or short circuits from lower strata sensorium apices to lower strata motorium apices. At the lowest stratum, these short-circuit connections are reflex actions. As we go up, we reach acquired, more complex skills which are almost built in like walking, sucking, grasping and so on. Further up we get early learned patterns, now pushed down below the level of consciousness. Further up still, we get more developed and complicated skills which have to be consciously learned and, later still, pushed down out of consciousness to a bypass connection. They no longer require the reinforcement of attention, but go forward automatically. As we go upwards, the apices elaborate and reach out more and more for wider and wider reference areas. At the top apical region, the brain deals with rarer types of event. That is why this mischievous, intrusive, unstoppable, adventurous, cowardly, generalist animal, Man, who pushed himself into so many unprovided for environments, had to develop the biggest cortex or final reference area at top level.

He had to store more information and find more ways of connecting and relating it. But, and this is the biggest but of all, by far the most important part of the process of living is the constant perception and reaction which is going on at lower unconscious levels. *Attention* is only needed for the rare, the strange, the unexpected, the new phenomenon. The vast majority of the activity in the brain happens probably in the subcortical regions. Only the rare, the flukey, the low probability event, has to be dealt with at the top cortical or conscious level. That is why they found, in those horrid experiments with cats, that even when the whole cortex had been removed the cat could still 'learn' simple lessons. With stimulus and reward having very high probability connections, it could still cope without its final, widest reference area.

The parallel in the social organization is this. To the big boss, the model says, if he does not know it already, bypass everything you can. Once new things are resolved, push responsibility down the network.

You will make people happier because they have brains and want to use them, and you will release yourself for your true function which is exploratory, relational, that of spreading out wider and wider nets of enquiry and experiment.

If you are efficient you are *not* running the firm. It is running itself. Your job is to watch for the unusual, to deal with a new combination, to correct things that go wrong and change the pattern of the flow of information where this goes wrong. Encourage bypasses, short-cuts, wherever they improve things. Reduce your informational load as much as you dare. The boss who says about a long report 'take it away and get it on one sheet of paper' has got the right idea. The boss who demands more and more and more detail has got the wrong idea. His job is to hire people who can deal with detail, not to deal with it himself *unless and until* something has gone wrong.

In an animal its boss, attention, can be concentrated on the tiniest detail of its input if some contradiction, problem or unusual event arises in connection with it. So should the boss, rarely, be on the factory floor looking at the bearings on the machine itself, and only then when the normal systems have broken down. The best motto for a manager that I know is 'work so as to make yourself unnecessary'. You will not succeed but you may free yourself to be a much better risk and opportunity taker. I advise strenuously against accumulation of unnecessary data. Keep communications short and do not memorandise the world and his wife. The attention paid to your paper work is inversely proportional to the amount of it. A further conclusion is, encourage people on the sales or input side to condense, summate and simplify information and try to arrange that the elaboration of instructions takes place at a number of stages in the works, rather than trying to make all decisions centrally and specifying too exactly the behaviour of people you do not know on the factory floor. That is the job of the strata of managers and foremen below you. They will do it better than you will and you will get less friction. Every workman is a polyhierarchic system in himself with built in randomness, learning ability. He knows his bit of the motorium better than anyone else. Make his foreman consult him and leave him some freedom of action. The higher you are in the firm, the further forward you should be looking, the bigger chances you should be taking, the lower the probabilities you will be dealing with and the better must be your skill at estimating them. Unless you have a high tolerance for insecurity, grasp of essentials, and a readiness to have most of your time wasted in unsuccessful exploratory activities, do not aspire to be a big boss. Your pay-offs are rarer but they are bigger. The best boss is a chance taker, but one who takes chances only at his own level and insists on higher probabilities at those below.

Most important of all, the boss must remember that he is in charge of a morphostat and that, whether he likes it or not, it will resist change at all points always. And this is not bad. As an innovator, I have had to work against this trend all my life. It is a good and healthy fight and I am a much better innovator for having had to wage it. No one but a madman welcomes change without strong prospect of advantage. Everyone has a right to question changes and any firm that is too suggestible to its innovators will prove to be too unstable. Fundamental innovations come only rarely from firmly established companies. A really new product usually brings out a new class of companies to deal with it. This is because surviving companies are morphostats. Having specialized for some niche in the economic network, they can rarely change fundamentally. This is as it should be, will be and must be. The job of a boss is firstly, primarily and mostly to hold together his team, to keep them happy. This will only be done by putting them into a relatively predictable system. But the boss must seize advantageous adaptions, moves towards metastability, improvements in change-resisting ability. As an organization grows, the boss will have to widen horizons and become more bosslike in the sense outlined in the paragraphs above. At the very top level of the largest organization problems are so big and unknowable that the boss must act on hunches, by the general feel, smell and sense of the situation. Whatever action he takes will have long, slow, unknowable consequences, most of which he will never see. The information that comes to him will have had to be so highly condensed and summated that it will be only a vague general sense of the situation that he can have. The boss can go down to sensorium, the interface and sample a few points, but that is the best he can do.

The Implications for Democracy and Law

Democracy. The trouble with democracy is that it has too few strata. People, representatives, cabinet, prime minister. Monohierarchic in appearance but polyhierarchic in fact. But it was not democracy that produced the polyhierarchic system. It grew like that because of the uncomprehended laws of information flow, unaffected by the voting. Democracy gives a binary choice of, effectively, a single person, prime minister or president every five years. To say that this is in the remotest sense the people expressing their wishes is the wallop of a whale-sized cod. It works, rough enough, because it gives the electorate the Power of the Boot, the chance to disturb the system enough to make the centre sensitive to the sensorium. But the real influence of the individual is with his consumer licences – money. Money flow changes the system. The hierarchy up which you send your money changes the whole industrial pattern. You pass it to a shopkeeper, who passes it to a wholesaler who passes it to a factory. Then it passes down through an opposite hierarchy of workmen. If enough of you change the pattern often enough the shape of the works will change because of your money votes.

The political force of deliberately-directed spending is a vast and potentially untapped power. On the motorium side new hierarchies, trade unions, have arisen because the proprioceptive feedback signals were too often ignored. The unions gathered strength and grew their own hierarchies and it was not until they did that that they were able to push back up their signals and affect the way things work. The consumer, alas, has only recently thought of getting organized. The commercial system may develop a consumer-organizing system which can make its weight felt. But if the result of this is simply a more consumerist society it will be worse than useless. Strikes at least have the merit of reducing overconsumption. We must hope that the Naders of this world will find that they can do more about the ecology problem than government, that the pressures of a new morality valid for a long term future for our species will one day influence the central decisions more than the pressure of either money or strikes.

Justice, Laws, Codes, Rules and Regulations

These are systems to create order by one stratum monohierarchic instruction. They come from one source and are supposed to apply equally to all. Usually they are a useful guide in the central semantic region but towards the borders of the classes described in them there are always the awkward 'border-line cases' where they create injustice. There are two forces demanding invariable regulation. Those in authority who are too lazy to consider evidence and make decisions demand computer-like programmes or codes and those who are ruled ask for the same because they feel more secure in a system where they 'know where they stand'. The industrial manager dealing with a particular case finds that he is unintentionally creating a kind of 'case law' and setting precedents which become shackles to future action. There is no law or code which does not go wrong at the borderline because there is no class in nature which has clean borderlines. In a truly polyhierarchic model where adequate indeterminacy is preserved at all points in the network we should see less flat invariable regulation and more decisions by people on the spot dealing with the particular case on its merits. We should see the best computer known in the universe, the human mind, used more and we should find it used especially and particularly in that function at which it excels, judgement.

Freedom

Freedom. As an industrial innovator by profession and a Socialist, liberal and progressive by inclination and early conviction, I found the general pattern of my conclusions as I reached them, extremely unpalatable. It seems likely that my crude attempt to create a viable generalist model upon which to restructure, conceptually, the information about living systems which is available, will be labelled as ultra-Conservative and even reactionary. But I must not draw back because of that. The bionic or biomorphic view I am advancing is a model, a hypothesis, a conceptual system for examination, appraisal, modification, acceptance or rejection. Ideas, models and hypotheses, are expendable and my responsibility is to communicate an idea which seems to me to be useful and which, as a human being, I feel I have a duty to pass on. I am convinced of its potential value, but the evaluation of the loosely-bound set of ideas I have put forward is the task of my readers and I wish them luck.

What I have said is not coherent in the sense that it is all untrue if one part is. My models can be useful and predictive in one sphere and not in another or in one respect and not in another. They are, I hope, like any biomorphic scheme for knowing the world, a corrigible first approximation, not an iron law awaiting falsification.

Ardrey in *Social Contract* wrote that in every species there was visible an imponderable aspect which he called 'identity'; the animal's insistence on being itself; its 'drive', or 'freedom of action'.

In humans, boss-prone though we are, the pressure for individual freedom is fiercely evident. In the West, we have built up a society for which the ultimate aim seems to be the achievement for every individual of the maximum personal freedom compatible with the continuation of the life-support system and with the freedom of other members. Building up our ordered stable systems, our organizations, we are both helped and hindered by the pressure at all levels by members to escape from the constraints of these very systems. Our desire for stability and security drives us as a species to regulate ourselves, but our contradictory desire for individual freedom urges us to break our own regulations. The apparent contradiction is resolved by the idea of learning. Learning involves experiment and experiment is a random input which is not determined by the environment but which comes from the exploratory necessities of the creature whose behaviour patterns are not built in, but reassembled, in each generation. If any organization, at any level, manages completely to suppress random variations then, at that level adjustment, learning by experience, has ceased. It will then only be a matter of time before some configuration of circumstances arises which will destroy the system. Our urge to be unique, indeterminate, is inbuilt and essential. Whim is a tool of life. In every individual, indeterminism is pushed towards the centre. It can never be eliminated from there, and this is as true of the organization. There are people, and it is important that there should be people, who will pursue some apparently irrational internal goal against all obvious conclusions. The cranks, oddities, outsiders, inventors, innovators and thinkers can be seen as sociological devices for injecting a random input into the social system. They are and must be expendable but they are and will always be essential as a set. It is their task to provide a wide range of experimental options which are essential to the continuation of morphostatic systems. The conclusions for an organization are that decision-making and freedom of action should be pushed as far down the network as possible. If, at any point in the network, a human being is working and not using his elaborate polyhierarchic decision-making system, then he is being wasted. The job can be done by a machine.

The human urge towards freedom is the driving force of those who regret the rigidities of a polyhierarchic system, bohemians, anarchists, hippies, drop-outs, artists, intellectuals, inventors, writers, poets . . .

Here my mind has misgivings. Is that all? Art cannot be seen to be morphostatic, biologically advantageous, yet, in man, it is ubiquitous and has been evident from his beginnings. There is surely something more here – something my hypothesis can do nothing with. Art seems to be one Good Thing where the biological advantage is unobvious. I can only remind the reader of an idea put forward by Eccles and subscribed to by Sir Cyril Burt. But such a *volte-face* justifies another chapter, and I shall deal with the matter later.

Anarchists

The original set of concepts from which communism grew are basically anarchistic. Marx, like Proudhon, Kropotkin and Malatesta felt quite sure, as I have said, that apart from villainous capitalists, priests, kings and other leaders, men are basically good and moral and capable of living in properly functioning groups without hierarchic leadership and 'institutions'.

Experience with anarchistic communes gives little grounds for faith in this pattern. In those that are successful and viable, closer examination shows at least one individual who has taken on the special role of ensuring the coherence of the group and that it meets its minimum corporate needs. The anarchist concept arises from a false view of the nature of people. There is nothing basically evil about the selfish, aggressive and predatory behavioural drives with which almost all human beings are equipped. Although he has been a social animal since he emerged as a separate species, Mankind arose from a predator and was originally evolved for a predatory life. It was upon this substrate that social life had to grow. The early symbiotic groups of humans had to evolve a cultural heredity to overcome the effect of their genetic heredity. They developed a power of suggestibility, proneness to accept instructions. They developed traditions, rituals, codes and moralities which inhibited and reduced the effect of their elementary drives, making it difficult for them to work together effectively.

The cooperative ensembles of men evolved cultural systems which themselves survived and grew. It would be nice if it were true that all men are basically good, where good means altruistic, unselfish. But it is evident that they are not. They have to struggle to contain, inhibit and prevent the drives developed for a more primitive form of life. Social behaviour, altruism are precarious, hard won virtues and will be for a few more million years until, by the slow process of genetic evolution, or more quickly by eugenic interference, the now redundant aggressive drives are reduced to vestiges. Probably already man is more pacific and moral than he was a half a million years ago. But genetics promises us only slow progress. I am afraid that the anarchists may have a long wait before their ideas can produce a healthy and effective society. The only grain of comfort I have for them is that the polyhierarchic model indicates that the monohierarchic structure of authority is wrong and misleading and that the formation of autonomic links is desirable. This means that large organizations will function more effectively if they delegate decision-making as far down both the networks as they can. Autonomic cross-links should be formed wherever possible in regions where overall strategy is not involved. For large societies to survive, they too must, when the problem is urgent, concentrate on one problem at a time. They must have an overall policy and a system of priorities and this requires a central decision-making centre where these priorities are decided. They must have the homologue of 'ego' and 'attention'. Its horrid name is 'boss'. 'Down with the boss', is merely the cry of self-announcement of a new boss. 'Down with the elite', can only be the birth-cry of a new-born élite.

Power and the Trappings of Power

People are obsessed by the idea of power. What is power in a morphostat? In human society, each person has two positions in the network: one as a receptor sending up need signals and the other as an effector doing a part of a job. We all have to take orders. Even the big boss is the slave of the system and much of what he has to do is dictated to him by his environmental input.

But this particular impudent animal, this species we belong to, is the one that never grew up, never stopped playing, it retained, even in the adult form, a bit of central freedom, freedom to choose between repertoires of established action patterns. We cling with great tenacity to this 'free will'. It is vital to us. We will die for it. So when we become an effector and have to take orders, we accept but we are always a little in revolt against them. Most men like the security of an authority-structure and clear instructions at first, but many gradually come to want more freedom of action and power of decision. In any morphostat, any non-equiponderous system, elements of the system have to accept instructions from other elements or the whole thing breaks down. Since humans are all alike in appearance, we have to find some way of making the effect of some greater than that of the others in certain roles. We have to create bosses. We used to put uncomfortable, spikey metal hats on them, and sit them on special chairs called thrones to show everybody that this was the one you took most notice of. Now we just write 'Manager' on the door of their offices and carpet their floors. Mostly we dress them differently and give them a bigger car or some other label, so that all members of the collectivity will understand where instructions come from and be able to sort out which information to take most notice of. In other words, which are their inputs and which are their outputs, which are their post-synaptic connections which are their pre-synaptic connections, as Penfield puts it. The post-synaptic instruction *receiving* unit, human, does not relish this much but has to get used to it. That is the way morphostats work. But he exists in a pecking order. Others beyond him will receive his signal, suitably varied by his own random input of free will, and, generally speaking, everyone 'knows where he is'. The system settles down. Remove power, make everyone equal, equiponderous, and you turn an organization into a horde or mob, a herd into a stampede, an animal into a corpse and a cell into chemicals.

So how do we allocate roles? They have to be allocated, one way or another. The most peaceable system is probably the best. Fairity, they say, is a rarity. There is no *fair* way. In authoritarian systems it is done simply by appointment. Aristocracy used a heredity of privilege, influential roles being bagged by an élite or privileged class.

Élites

An élite is the name we give to a set in society whose signals are amplified to have big effects upon what happens. In highly-organized societies we cannot do without élites.

We have been looking not at the people but at the movement of information between points or gates in the network, roles. What of the incumbents of these roles? Having sketched our necessary network should we drop people in the role-holes at random? This would be an offshoot of the Rousseau doctrine of equality. It asserts that anyone, especially if he is anti-authority, uneducated, untrained and stupid, is equal in performance to anyone else. The wide pattern of religions and other beliefs shows that the human mind, when put to it, is capable of believing anything. But this particular faith remains a very special feat of credulity. In my opinion the principal difference between the over-developed countries and the overdevelop*ing* countries is that in one part of the world a social system grew up with a philosophy of the best man for the job. The role-holes in the social network have to be occupied. Those near the central decision apices need to be occupied by the best brains going. In the social system each node or locus is a whole polyhierarchic network in itself and we need to use at the centre those whose ability can work best for the rest of humanity. But if the élites contend for position and replace each other, the competition is good and healthy.

Our role allocation system, which has been too successful has been the competitive capitalist system in which boss roles are competed for on the basis of the best man for the job. Which really means a long bitter, but restrained struggle for power. The only other thing I can think of is using scientific methods but I wonder if psychometrics has reached the point yet. It is moving that way. It can certainly help if supplemented by a trial and error check as the work proceeds. A large complex society has to allocate highly-specified roles to everybody except a handful of parasites and pensioners and over-rewarded plutocrats. Chop it how you will, that is how it will come down and there is no way out. I have scanned the system and worked at all levels from labourer to Managing Director and I see no undisputed way of allocating boss-roles. One solution to the role-allocation problem was suggested by both Wells and Shaw: An egalitarian society, where role was separated from reward. But the end of that line is conscription. The present system shoos people into roles by a mixture of carrot and stick. Roles, where the right type of incumbent is in short supply, attract incumbents by increasing the size of the carrot.

There is another system with much merit and that is 'honour', the kind of insubstantial reward which costs society nothing and consists in certain attitude towards the incumbent of the role which pleases him and does not hurt us. It is an excellent system which should be made more use of. Unfortunately, the academics have messed it up in the intellectual field by their own self disgust and anti-intellectualism, so that it is no longer felt to be an honourable thing to be a university lecturer or professor, which is a pity. Many liberals and lefties have thrown out the baby – of honour, distinction, acclaim, fame and all the other socially-cheap inducements to social action – with the bath-water of hereditary privilege which certainly deserved to go. Now we are in a right old muddle with effort, ability, value, rare talent being offered smaller and smaller carrots both of the insubstantial 'honour' type and of the substantial 'money' type, while the economically powerful (when united) performers of simple tasks, which, for all their many virtues are in 'long supply' are being over-rewarded relative to contribution. We have not a meritocracy but a strikeocracy. If we keep on that way, the system will break down. But humanity is a morphostat. We shall not keep on that way.

Social Reward

The basis of the capitalist system was, as I have said, a more equitable system of social reward than that which prevailed before. Despite its manifest injustices and imbalance, it has the virtue, admitted even by its opponents, of creating more efficient methods of production leading to a more comfortable life in that part of the world where it has operated effectively.

The side-effect disadvantages are now apparent and the present rate of accelerating unnecessary industrial 'growth' and the forced unnecessary increase in consumption has to be eased to a halt.

Any org has to provide for the support of all its members and must have at its disposal a reward-punishment system to elicit cooperative behaviour. Propaganda, honours, preferment, fame, respect, clear conscience, luxury; as well as fines, prison, condemnation, dismissal are some of the behaviour-changing mechanisms of society.

The capitalist system relies theoretically almost entirely on money and imprisonment as its pleasure/pain system and this has manifest disadvantages. Much antisocial behaviour is highly rewarded. And good financial guesswork is over-rewarded too!

Money, a motor signal

The flow of money is an indicator of the direction of the flow of information. Money flows from the instructor (employer) to the instructed (employed). It is received by the citizen in his role as a producer or subordinate and passed on by him in his role as a consumer or beneficiary of the activities of society. We could describe it as a licensed *need* signal. The individual elements of human society have many needs which have to be satisfied. Neither the society nor the organizations which form part of it can satisfy all the needs and aspirations, at all times, of all its members. We need a way to select – from among need signals so that the system shall not be brought to a halt by their plethora. Money is a limited licence to command. In most societies, broadly speaking, it is used as a means of inducing patterns of individual behaviour required for the continuance of society and its organizations. The route money takes through the afferent hierarchies decides, on balance, the amount of activity which will be generated from the apical decision centres in the offices of the manufacturing organizations. Its flow takes exactly the same pattern as the flow of information. It is polyhierarchic. It comes from a base of consumers, converges upon an apical array of centres of instructions, factories, local government offices, government itself and from these centres it diverges hierarchically until it is distributed to the same array of citizens in their role as producers. The fact that money can take the form of metal and paper artifacts, marks on paper in a bank or differences in magnetism on a computer tape, makes it clear that it is informational in nature. It passes the test of information. It can be transduced into numerous coded forms without losing its semantic content. It is beyond the scope of this book to follow the complexities of its flow and the complications of our world monetary system. I have indicated a way of looking at it; it may help us a little in understanding and prediction.

Within organizations there is the flow of money to the members which is organized by the top management and in this sense it is an additional excitatory input. But it is only this in a long term view. Its role in the leadership process is much less than is usually imagined. The stability (security) seeking efforts of employees eventually have the effect of levelling out variations in the money flow so that its rewarding effect is gradually diminished. In some senses it is the analogue of the blood supply in the animal brain. However it is used by bosses as one of the tools in his behaviour-changing toolkit. Fortunately for all the bosses in the world, mankind is a boss-prone animal. Every human is brought up in a family in which he learns to be suggestible to information coming from certain humans, his parents. A society of animals without an inbuilt tendency to throw up leaders and accept leadership would stand little chance in a competitive situation against more organizable animals. A species which can form functioning societies, consisting of a symbiotic pattern of cooperating organizations, needs both a great majority of relatively suggestible members and a small minority of self-directed and bossy members. In Humanity, the problem is solved by the existence, either built-in or acquired, of two modalities of behaviour. Most people can switch quite easily from leader to follower roles according to their assigned place in the particular group they happen to be with. The leader/follower system is basic, but money is a useful amplifier. But as a method of social reward the money system is breaking down.

The underlying theory was that the entrepreneur, inventor, businessman, who risked his money and time in building up more efficient ways of producing goods and services to satisfy the needs of humanity should be rewarded for this by an especially large issue of consumption licences. The effect of this was supposed to reinforce those activities which were popular, *i.e.* the manufacture of those goods and services which were greatly required or valued by men, and so the system was supposed to create a better and better fit of the supply profile to the profile presented by the requirements, demands, needs of the individual members of society.

The system is breaking down because the central aspect of the system, which was most important, is that the entrepreneur could use money to stimulate the appropriate type of behaviour in other people by paying them. The reward was to be in accordance with the value of the service, the amount of intelligence required to perform it, the reliability of the worker and the difficulty and complication of the task. This was the theory and it worked for a time, partially.

Under the influence of Marxism, however, there grew up the Socialist and Trade Union movements. They gained impetus from the great inequalities of the distribution of money which resulted in the free operation of the described system. Workers organizations have ameliorated the harshness of the capitalist system and gradually undermined the ability of the boss to reward employees in accordance with his own valuation of their service. In doing this, they have been whittling away at the 'behaviour-changing' power or learning aspect at the motorium of a polyhierarchic system. The polyhierarchic structures, called trade unions, have achieved a bargaining power in society which operates in independence, as it were, of the sensory input because they have grown up at the motor interface. The consumer is constantly paying higher prices for the same goods, because of demands that he himself is making on society as a producer. The individual human in his producer role is kicking his own arse in his consumer role. The result is upsetting the capitalist pattern of distribution of wealth, basically a meritocracy, and causing the storms, tides and instabilities of the money situation in the world.

These problems, as far as we can see, do not seem to affect the Socialist world. Here a rigid, firm, meritocratic system rules. However, the Communist systems, despite its unhierarchic model, unsuccessfully trying to be monohierarchic. The self-organizing element in capitalist society is missing so that the supplies of goods and services available to individuals are poorer and less various than they are in the more advanced countries. Also the profile of supply has a worse fit to that of needs and aspirations.

What is needed is a more scientific reward and punishment system, based on a profile of goals, that is a morality valid for the whole of humanity in the longest possible view.

If there is to be any chance of achieving the enormous behaviour changes which will be required if humanity is to survive, in any sensible fashion, on this planet, we shall have to have a better system of social reward and punishment. Ideas are two a penny and so I would like to throw in my ha'p'orth. The science of psychometrics and the business of advertising, publicity and opinion manipulation are now relatively well advanced. We are beginning to be able to tell sufficiently well what people's capabilities are both as to intelligence and as regards many other factors of personality and we are also able to persuade people into great changes in behaviour patterns. The rise of Hitler in Germany, the success of purveyors of poisons, like tobacco and alcohol, in foisting their products on to the public, testify to this in a negative way. On the other hand, the very rapid increase in the awareness of ecological problems recently shows the positive power that is available to be used if only we can find a way to do it.

It is no use telling anyone like me, who was around during the second world war, that 'people don't change'. We saw whole nations change absolutely, their habits of work, their consumption and their social behaviour in the course of a few months. The changes needed now can be made but there is little trend that way so far. Later this century, when the shoe pinches a little tighter, we may see more action, but preparation is needed now.

I would like to see a new profession, a set of dedicated professionals specializing in the problems of social reward and punishment. Abandoning the fear of 'manipulation' they would be frankly aiming at changing behaviour. Their work would range from penology to making decisions about who should occupy high-ranking posts in government. They would have to be as reliable and trusted as judges are in our present legal system and would have to be, and be seen to be, completely incorruptible. Perhaps the technique, curiously called Social Engineering is the beginning we need here.

A Biomorphic View of Pure Science

In the biomorphic view there is no such thing as Pure Science. Science is the sensory system of Mankind as a whole. The examations of the sensory input for any org, vary along a spectrum of generality, and probability of relevance. All are exploratory and therefore have a probability of relevance (of reaching through to the decision centres and generating motor activity), of less than one. Some exploratory activity has a very low probability of pay-off and we must then expect the pay-off to be very high for it to be worth the effort. Other exploratory activity has a very high probability of pay-off and we may therefore be content with a relatively small pay-off.

On this spectrum Pure Science is directed towards uncovering extremely general regularities in the universe which have very wide applicability and therefore very great value in many fields. Accordingly we can afford to expend a very great deal in fundamental investigations of this kind without seeing very clearly how and where the applications will arise. At the other end of the spectrum we move from science to technological development and here the probability of advantage must become much higher; often so high that we can calculate the cost/benefit advantage of the developmental activity in positive terms. The saddest thing about the underlying morality of science is that so much of the cachet and self-value has been attached to the pure scientist and so little to the, much more often much more useful, applied scientist who actually delivers the goods. The result has been, an over concentration on Pure Science. The best minds are attracted into the fields where the greater part of the activity is by the very nature of the problems destined to be wasted. The position of the teacher, the man who actually talks to students, is also far too low in the academic peck order. Those who have too much to do with students are looked down upon by their research colleagues. This is one more indication that the scientist has forgotten that his main raison d'être is that of communication.

The Scientists

Scientists, by and large are out of touch and, like other social divisions, they have made a 'badge of difference' out of their own private language. Like the hippies they are proud of their failure to communicate. The honoured 'pure' scientist is really at a humble level, at the observation sensorium of the org humanity. Science is good because it is relatively international and transcends most other boundaries. But a sensorium with no connections to the motorium via the apical regions is useless. If the apical decision centres do not get the message and act on it, then the whole pack and boiling of scientists are a waste of talent, time and money.

But it is not the scientist's problem. What is missing is the polyhierarchic intercommunications network between him and the decision centres.

Under the drive of the Territorial Imperative, each scientist instinctively defends his own little arc of the advancing circle of knowledge. As new men crowd in, the arcs are divided, subdivided and divided again. Each man defends his territory and fights off intruders and outsiders like me. The message is 'ignore those who don't know the language, do not try to find out what they are getting at'. One man looked at an early version of my ideas here for two years. At the end of it he told me he was 'embarrassed' by my 'solecisms' and 'unusual language'. He made no attempt to evaluate the idea or see if perhaps I had a point. You, dear reader, must be the judge as to whether he did the right thing. By his standards, and those of most academics, he certainly did. On the other hand, one or two academics, Professor Andresky, Professor R. T. Green, Professor Sir Cyril Burt, Professor John Good *have* listened to and encouraged me, and that is one reason why I dare to utter at all. But back to my onions after the gossip.

Scientists despise popularizers like Bronowski, Ardrey, Morris and Eysenck. They are rejected and objected to because they are the 'scabs' of the scientific world. They do not hide away behind the normal academic facade, the mock humility, abhorrence of publicity, and obscurity of language. In fact, they are doing great service in creating the communication link, which is so essential, between science and the decision centres. If science is not communication, it is nothing. Science could be defined as a rigorous investigation of what is communicable between brains. Science transmits the regularities of the universe. Due to the inefficiencies of monolinear communication, it cannot be very good at it. But still it is the best we have. I have a nice story about the obscurity of language of those who are doing seminal thinking in the very field I am writing in.

A man called Wilfred Hyde wrote three articles in the Mensa Journal about the functioning of the brain. Many members wrote to me to say they could not understand a single word and wondered if he was not just talking gobbledy-gook. My own brief reading (after many years speculation in the same field) was that Hyde did have some insight but he was definitely not trying very hard to communicate it.

However, independently of me, Professor Fremlin of Birmingham University tested a personal theory by writing him a carefully phrased letter, in gobbledy-gook, posing some questions. He got a completely straight-faced answer which took the letter, or appeared to do, completely seriously. Personally I would like to see a public debate between the two. The whole thing might be a lesson in the necessity for scientists to communicate, or at least to be seen to be trying to do so. My final message to the scientists is this. If you have failed to communicate, you have failed, period. Your work is useless, you are wasting your time and our money. A test of your usefulness is whether you change decisions at the decision centres. If not, you are a flop but do not worry, adventurers, explorers, scientists and scouts waste most of their time. We cannot demand a hundred per cent pay-off. Scientists, like intellectuals, are expendable. It is not given to us to know which bits will pay off, but we ought to be working to some strategy of probability estimating in expending resources. We should also fight hard against the institutionalization of science. It is the enemy of everything that science ought to be. Institutions are orgs and defend themselves as orgs whether they are useful or not. Once set up, a scientific establishment will go on probing deeper and deeper into the minutinae of a subject long past the point where the law of diminishing returns makes their activity wasteful. This kind of thing should be ruthlessly curtailed because we need more brains at the decision centres and not so many down at the sensorium. We should remove the 'honour' from the 'pure' scientists and push it back up to the higher regions, the interface between science and the motorium, where scientific discoveries advantageously change human behaviour.

It is from the scientist that we must expect the ultimate guidance on the basic ecological problems which confront us but it is the strata that transduce the information into instructions that are lacking.

Universities

Many advanced civilizations in the past developed cultural centres which attracted intelligent and informed people from wide areas. Out of their interaction many good things arose. These centres acted as a repository and a transmission system for the cultural inheritance of information, ideas and speculations. When writing appeared, the effect of these interactions became cumulative and transmissible through the generations.

The modern development of this trend is great and ubiquitous. Universities proliferate and a perceptible proportion of the population has become an academic establishment whose livelihood and comforts are provided by the societies in which they function.

Any cost/benefit exercise on the value of Universities to humanity must, at least on short-term, give a positive picture because of the great contribution that they have made to the quality of human life in many spheres. But it would be foolhardy to claim that this cost/benefit ratio is unimprovable. The rate of expansion in numbers, size, population and in cost of Universities has been exponential and that kind of curve leads to pessimistic assumptions about the cost/benefit advantage. In the absence of clear evidence, the initial assumption should be that investment of this kind is subject to the law of diminishing returns and the advantage to humanity from this activity is moving asymptotically towards zero.

The least we can say is that this is a very valid question, well worth examination. There are, of course, very many human activities of a very much less beneficial type of which the same might be said. These also should be investigated, perhaps with priority. But as the world moves towards a future of frugality which at this point seems inevitable, we must not rule out, *ab initio*, that some of the axes of economy may have to be carried into the groves of Academe. It may be that we shall need to have more students and scientists who pursue their calling for the love of it and less who make a profession of it.

There are few who would deny that the activities in Universities are good, moral and desirable. But many might deny that science is best conducted by scientific establishments or that study, meditation, speculation and experiment, exciting, fascinating and all-absorbing as they are to many people, need necessarily receive the additional reward of a leisured, unpressured and relatively affluent life with a reduced contribution. Scientific papers and periodicals are ground out faster and faster in an academic rat-race and packed away systematically into inaccessibility in choked libraries. The proportion of researches that have any effect whatsoever on the life of men becomes smaller and smaller. The effort expended relative to the result achieved gets less and less. Somewhere there must be a limit.

The Academic Iconoclasts

Among the growing army of academics is one unhappy sub-set which is infected by the idea of the 'noble savage' by Equipotential Equiponderous Man and dialectical materialism. They sincerely think that the 'State' must 'wither away', and feel they should help the process. They project an attitude of resistance to all visible leadership, establishment or authority. They are ashamed to find themselves able to think, reason and solve problems better than others because this is at variance with the model. Having equal rights, equal intelligence, equal ability, each should have equal opportunities and equal effect on outcomes.

Confronted with the awkward fact that people do not conform to the model, their love for humanity closes their eyes to the evidence that inequalities of ability between people may be innate. They search ever closer and closer to the moment of conception for environmental reasons for the difference.

Conclusive studies with uniovular twins have shown that only about 20-30 per cent of the variance in mental ability can be accounted for by environmental factors but the evidence is easily dismissed because of its lack of correspondence with the model. Confused by the mismatch between the Marxist model and the facts, this particular set of the academics has, in perfect sincerity, contributed to the widespread unrest, disaffection and rejection of cultural tradition which seems to be affecting students in most parts of the world.

Completely abandoning that important part of their role that of transmitters of advantageous cultural data, information, practices and disciplines, these sad, ashamed academics have infected a whole generation of students with a negative attitude towards the very positive activities of study, intellectuality, disciplined investigation, and scholarship itself.

The very word intellectual has become an insult and the respect in which a scholar and teacher was once held has been lost because the world has accepted the views of some academics about themselves. Students have been taught that equality and justice can only be achieved by a sort of apocalyptic Death and Resurrection of the Whole System: Revolution. But the nasty, bloody, painful, horrid and uncomfortable experiment has been tried enough. Where it has been tried it has in every case, been rejected. A many level, ostensibly monohierarchic but really polyhierarchic system, has been torn down and immediately there has been chaos until another has been erected in its place. The rigidity and the authoritarianism has been more, not less after the revolution than it was before. The marxist communist model has never even been tried. Revolution has been the seizure of power from one élite by another élite, often very much more monohierarchic than the first. Only gradually do Communist revolutionary governments settle down into the necessary polyhierarchic mode. As they do they become more efficient. But their retention of central strategic control gives them an advantage. They have it because they are not more but less communistic in the early sense of the word. The State did not wither away. It grew tough, strong, and entrenched.

My main hope is that the World Brain, the communication system of the super org which is organizing itself on the biomass of the world may become conscious and develop connections with the World Motorium in time.

The trend is there. Polyhierarchic international centres are developing. I count over fifteen hundred international organizations in the 1964/5 Year Book and probably not all are entered. There would appear to be some need for further strata above these apices but their spontaneous formation is the beginning of the necessary process.

Mensa, the Ubiquitous University

I myself helped to build one of these – Mensa. A collectivity of people of above average intelligence, which is, as far as we can extend it, international and polypolitical (rather than apolitical). It has no dogma and its aim is to transcend the mental boundaries which divide humanity. Mensans feel that if there is any section of humanity which is able to surmount, or at least peep over, political, ideological, religious, cultural, racial, social and occupational divisions it is the intelligent.

'What would happen', we asked, 'if we built up an association around the ability to comprehend rather than around the blind acceptance of some dogma?' Some of us dreamed of an élite, not of privilege but of service. A final cross-reference communication region where there can be an interplay of ideas leading to the cross fertilization that may be needed to find the perhaps unlikely combinations of activity which will solve the problems that man's brain has created in the biosphere.

Since the world is in great need of the services of its more able occupants and since people are naturally suspicious of privilege and power I would like to see the able people of the world visibly reject both so that they may gain influence and so that the interaction of their investigations, their imagination, and speculations may be the better able to produce solutions of the problems.

Even more important is the problem of setting goals. The present codes and moralities represent the success and failure signals at the social level. Most of them have been derived from dogmatic religions or ideologies and were not conceived in the light of a world civilization.

The task of the intellectual of tomorrow, and perhaps Mensa can play a humble part, is to produce that set of moral imperatives which is valid for all humanity, long term. The World Org needs a success measuring system and a means of transmitting its messages to the decision centres. This, more than the exercise of power seems to me to be the function of those who, through no virtue in them, have been born with the power to comprehend. False modesty and simulated humility has no place here. It is a cop out.

Chapter 11 World Org

ON THE SUBSTRATE, individual men and women, there has grown an elaborate territorial pattern of organizations, nations, which have fixed geographical boundaries. Between them they cover the surface of the planet as far as it is able to support human life. These nations have developed relatively recently out of the coalescence or conquest of a pattern of smaller territorial organizations, kingdoms and tribal areas. From time to time in the past six thousand years there have been brief periods of civilization when large nations and even empires grew from a successful organizational pattern starting at a small centre. Until the last few hundred years they were all, at least in external form, mono-hierarchic with a system of regional delegation made necessary by slow communications. But there existed within each a source of arousal which could bring them into a warlike, a fully cooperative mode for purposes of aggression or defence. But parallel with this structure of conquest and territorial seizure and simultaneously with it there was a radiation and interaction of cultural and technical information and gradually, after small beginnings, a trading system grew up which was coextensive with and pervaded much of the pattern of kingdoms. With the growth and strengthening of this pattern of independent traders, or culture-, technique-, know-how-mongers, a sketchy network of world communications was set up. It was trading more than war which led to the maritime exploration of the world.

The activity of the traders, later of manufacturers and later still of scientists, was, in fact, the visible appearance of a system which was at first polycentric and later polyhierarchic. The territorial bosses, the kings of the medieval system at first resisted the independent trading activities but gradually the advantages were seen to be much greater than the loss of control involved.

The satisfaction of human needs was being delegated to subsidiary decision centres and the pattern of organization was becoming poly-hierarchic. The system that has been called capitalism is in fact a poly-hierarchic system. Even its opponents have paid tributes to its success, but the citizens of the world and particularly the workers who now came under the control of untraditional rulers, people of a very different stamp from the hereditary cast of warriors they had accepted for so long, began to revolt against this new, unfamiliar pattern.

What the Socialists and Communists were asking for was an even greater extension of the same system; for the system to become more polyhierarchic, so much so that there should be as many decision centres as there are people. They, the reformers, were asking for anarchism. But the Communist movement, born under the impetus of the universal appetite for 'freedom', produced, in fact, a system which was merely a return to the normally monohierarchic system which had been superseded by an improved polyhierarchic one.

Despite Communism, however, the network of commercial and trading information became ubiquitous, it transcended all frontiers and now has its effect everywhere. Simultaneously with the growth of the communications network of commerce, other polyhierarchic networks developed. Science became international and ubiquitous. Cultural associations, religions, social work agencies, medicine, every discipline and every functional grouping developed an international communications system. A polyhierarchic world system of communications developed in many fields.

Today the Communist world is integrating itself ever more fully into the system.

Communications between the two worlds, the Capitalist and Communist one, were at first limited by the monohierarchic pattern in the Communist world but gradually a richer and richer system of low level contacts has grown up so that the inefficiencies and informational problems of the monohierarchic system are largely avoided by a growing net of bypasses.

While the politicians have been talking about it, the human inhabitants of the world have become an org. Mankind has developed an informational network which links all men into a tenuous but definite symbiotic whole. This process has been called progress, but it has no affinity with evolutionary progress. Evolutionary progress is competitive, with more divergent morphostatic forms, surviving better. This process, the feeling-out and growing together of separate orgs into a super-org is emergent and *convergent.* It is something strange and new. The politicians who are arguing for 'World State' are wasting their time. It is here. The only problem is that the political structures have not yet been adapted to it.

The links are not yet very strong. The separate regions and areas are semi-independent. They are, here and there, capable of schizophrenic conflict, but all evidence points to the fact that the volume of world communications is expanding at an exponential rate. Unless the trend is reversed, then the whole world of men will soon be united by a rich communications network. The totality of human behaviour everywhere in the world will become the outcome of the totality of information generated everywhere in the world. It may take the politicians and national leaders a generation or two to discover the fact, but the reality is here. It is all happening.

World Plan

The idea of a large-scale plan for a whole society arose first in the socialist world. The ideological basis of Communism leads to the idea that a National Plan would work itself out by the interaction of 'the Masses without Capitalist Exploiters'. Now the Western world has taken over the idea and everyone accepts the 'le planification' as the French say.

Large plans must be strategic, not tactical. But a semi-competitive structure of separate national plans is no substitute for a World Plan to continue our World Civilization. If the polyhierarchic communications network which has grown up on the substrate of man on earth is to ensure the continuing existence of the species, then the whole configuration of activity on the whole World Motorium will have to be changed radically. If the conclusions of the M.I.T. 'World Three' programme, the Club of Rome and other groups are even partially correct, then the world org is already receiving that input information which gives strong evidence that we are lurching towards a very great danger and a sharp ecological setback. Most intelligent people in the world are now aware of the dangers. But the world org lacks a conative centre an appetitive or goal setting or world morality input. And it lacks a success measuring input also. Social reward and social punishment are too little related to the long-term stability of the world org of human societies.

Though my conclusions lead me to some justification for Conservatism or at least for the more fashionable euphemism, conservationism, I have no real comfort for the traditionalists. I am not alarmed at the accelerating rate of change because of the *nature* of the change, it is in fact accelerating *progressive* change. I am alarmed because the advantages are short-term advantages. The problem for the politicians of the future is to preserve as much as possible of the comfort, leisure and pleasure of our style of life without stealing the very basis of life from our descendents. This generation of those who comprehend, the intelligent, must accept the uninstructed proxy of the unborn and provide the world not only with more generations but with a chance for them to live as well as possible. Frugality must be re-established as morally good and overbreeding and dysgenic breeding must be seen to be immoral. This still leaves room for a very good life.

Scattered there somewhere at the central apices in many countries and international offices are the decision centres where triggers must be pulled to switch humanity into a viable mode. At the moment there does not seem to be even the remotest chance that the central connecting system can grow out to contact these points and trigger them. Yet I believe it will and in its minute way, the writing of this book might be part of the process. I repeat, we shall not pray our way out of our problems nor shall we solve them by Gut-Thinking, Self Determination, Each Fulfilling his True Self, Freedom, Opting Out, Revolution, Goodwill, Warmheartedness, Kindliness or General Morality. We shall have, painfully, to Think Our Way Out. Humanity has become a whole despite itself. We shall survive together or collapse and die together. We cannot turn to kindly old Mother Nature to solve the problem either. We can only let her take over again after we have smashed up the system. The painfully slow process of evolutionary learning, one generation per lesson, does not operate within a symbiotic cooperating system. The world information system cancels evolution. Broadly and generally, the societies and individuals on earth are no longer competing all out. They are competing formally within a system of many constraints. The evolution of institutions has come to an end.

The World Brain, not yet come to consciousness, operating dreamlike, in a trance, is, autonomically, at least temporarily in charge. As things look today it will fail disastrously to solve the problem it has unconsciously taken on and this civilization will collapse early in the next century. But *that* statement which is now being made ubiquitously, in various ways, is a factor in the situation and it is not equivalent to all other statements. It is a powerful statement which may have a powerful effect. The amplification factor of a biological communication system is almost infinite. I said that the first operation of intelligence that we know of in the universe was that in the gradually changing information lines, chromosomes, in the individual cell. Second-order intelligence developed in thinking, and intelligence was exercised within each generation by animals with individual brains. Genetic evolution improved these brains until third-order thinking began to take place in organizations which had their own morphostatic control systems and on the substrate of men these organizations evolved the new style of heredity, cultural heredity; while they remained in competition the process of selection continued. But now they are coalescing into a single symbiotic whole. Now mankind is taking over the role of that filthy, cruel, vindictive, slovenly, slut, Kindly Old Mother Nature. For a little while we have a chance to show her that we can do a better job. Time is not on our side. She is waiting in the wings if we should fail.

Afterword **Tinkering with the Works**

I HAVE SAID THAT any morphostat must evolve a predictive brain, *i.e.* must rearrange the connections in its brain, so that it is an optimum predictive homologous model of the outside universe. It must be free (that means, must have regulated input of randomness) to rearrange those connections by successive approximations until the correspondence is *adequate for its purposes.* An encoded representation of reality in a brain which is an exact homologue of 'the world' is forever and obviously unobtainable. *Truth* is not for us. But models can be true *enough.*

In a universe where everything is predetermined there is no freedom, no randomness, to select from. A morphostat cannot try out and find by trial and error which encoded models of the universe are most predictive; if there is no input of randomness to permit variation of the model. Now there *is*, as Heisenberg proved, an input of randomness at the microcosmic level. We know that events at that level can affect cells because radiation, which consists of individual photons of energy can and does cause mutations and cancer, *i.e.* macroscopic change in a cell and then a soma. Now the behaviour of photons individually is indeterminate. So the random input which we require to understand learning by experience, might come from the microcosmic level. In this case we could look upon the brain as a way of amplifying the uncertainty of the microcosmic world so as to produce mass action in the mesocosm. Eccles suggested that this solves the problem of free will versus determinism. Morphostats can act against the weight of statistical pressure in an apparently determinist causal universe when uncertain microcosmic events are amplified by the subtle triggers within a cell and the elaborating uncertainty-amplifying system of a communication hierarchy. Thus it is suggested that the basic indeterminism of the universe can be amplified to show as free will or whim in man.

And a further suggestion by Eccles should be noted. Christianity posits a God, all-seeing, all knowing and all powerful. If he is, he must be either a sadist or incompetent but a God who is all-seeing and all-knowing but bound by statistical laws is a tenable but unprovable hypothesis. Eccles suggests that the only trigger this 'God' has to get at the physical universe, is where indeterminism-amplifying systems are built up so that he can get at the mesacosm via microcosm triggers.

Some biologists have tried to calculate the chances against the building up of the elaborate life patterns on earth on a hypothesis of the selection of chance occurrences and have been somewhat puzzled at the apparent length of the odds against it. If Eccles is right, maybe there has been some tinkering at the works. Perhaps the random input is not *quite* random so maybe the Maxwell demon is not a demon at all but the Life Force or God.

Bibliography

ALT, F. L. and RUBINOFF, M. (Editors): *Advances in Computers*, Vol 6, New York, Academic Press, 1965.

ANDRZEJEWSKI, S.: *Military Organisation and Society*, London, Routledge & Kegan Paul, 1954.

ARDREY, R.: *The Territorial Imperative*, London, Collins, 1967.

ARKAD'EV, A. G. and BRAVERMAN, E. M.: *Teaching Computers to Recognise Patterns*, London, Academic Press, 1967.

ASHLEY MONTAGU: *Human Heredity*, New York, Mentor, 1959.

BARTON, A. W.: *A Text Book on Heat*, London, Longmans, 1963.

BEER, S.: *Cybernetics and Management*, London, E.U.P., 1968.

BERELSON, B. and STEINER, G. A.: *Human Behaviour: An Inventory of Scientific Findings*, New York, Harcourt, Brace & World, 1964.

BELL, D.: *Decision Trees in Pattern Recognition*, National Physical Laboratory, D.T.I.

BERGSON, H.: *Matter and Memory*, London, Allen & Unwin, 1911.

CATTELL, R. B.: *Abilities: Their Structure, Growth and Action*, Boston, Houghton Mifflin, 1971.

CATTELL, R. B.: *Beyondism*, Oxford, Pergamon, 1972.

CHARDIN, P. T. de: *The Phenomenon of Man*, London, Fontana Books, 1965.

COHEN, J.: *Living Embryos*, Oxford, Pergamon, 1967.

CULBERTSON, J. T.: *Consciousness and Behaviour*, Dubuque, W. C. Brown & Co., 1950.

DARLINGTON, C. D.: *The Evolution of Man in Society*, London, Allen & Unwin, 1969.

DARLINGTON, C. D.: *Genetics and Man*, London, Pelican, 1966.

GOOD, I. J. (Editor): *The Scientist Speculates: An Anthology of Partially Baked Ideas.*

GREGORY, R. L.: *Eye and Brain*, London, Weidenfeld & Nicolson, 1966.

GREGORY, R. L.: *The Intelligent Eye*, London, Weidenfeld & Nicolson, 1970.

GUILDFORD, J. P.: *The Nature of Human Intelligence*, New York – London, McGraw Hill, 1967.

HAYEK, F. A.: *The Sensory Order*, London, Routledge & Kegan Paul, 1952.

HEBB, D. A.: *Organisation of Behaviour*, Chichester, Wiley, 1949.

HOOK, S. (Editor): *Dimensions of Mind*, London, Collier – Macmillan, 1961.

HUNTER, M. L.: *Memory*, London, Pelican, 1957.
KANAL, L. N.: *Pattern Recognition*, Washington D.C., Thompson Book Co.
KOESTLER, A.: *The Act of Creation*, London, Hutchinson, 1969.
LLOYD, B.: *Perception and Cognition*, London, Penguin.
LORENZ, K.: *On Aggression*, London, Methuen, 1966.
MACWORTH, J. E.: *Vigilance and Attention*, Harmondsworth, Penguin, 1970.
MACMILLAN, R. H. (Editor): *Nonlinear Control Systems Analysis*, Oxford, Pergamon, 1962.
MICHIE, D. (Editor): *Machine Intelligence I*, Edinburgh University Press, 1971.
MICHIE, D. (Editor): *Machine Intelligence II*, Edinburgh University Press, 1971.
MUSES, C. A.: *The Aspects of the Theory of Artificial Intelligence*, New York, Plenum Press, 1962.
NATHAN, P.: *The Nervous System*, London, Pelican, 1969.
PASK, G.: *An Approach to Cybernetics*, London, Hutchinson, 1961.
PENFIELD, W. and ROBERTS, L.: *Speech and Brain Mechanisms*, Princeton University Press, 1959.
PORTER, A.: *Cybernetics Simplified*, London, E.U.P., 1969.
ROSS ASHBY, W.: *Design for a Brain*, London, Chapman & Hall, 1960.
SAPARINA, Y.: *Cybernetics within us*, London, Central Books, 1966.
SAWYER, W. W.: *The Search for Pattern*, London, Pelican, 1970.
SOMMERHOFF, G.: *Analytical Biology*, O.U.P., 1950.
UHR, L. (Editor): *Pattern Recognition, Learning and Thought*, Chichester, Wiley, 1973.
UTTLEY, A. M.: *The Informon*, Journal of Theoretical Biology, 1970. 27. 31-67.
WIENER, N.: *Cybernetics: or Control and Communication in the Animal and Machine*, London, M.I.T. Press, 1961.
WRIGHT, Q.: *A Study of War*, University of Chicago Press, 1965.
WOOLRIDGE, D. E.: *The Machinery of the Brain*, London, McGraw-Hill, 1963.
YOUNG, J. F.: *Cybernetics*, London, Iliffe, 1969.

Index

Abnegation of responsibility 112
Academics 7, 166
Acausal 44
Acausality 95
Adaptive changes 40
Adler 108
Afferent 48, 49, 61, 62, 76, 77, 81, 89, 91, 100, 101, 125, 136, 139, 143, 146, 149, 160
Age of reason 112, 113
  of technology 112
Aleksander 79
Albrow 79
Alignment 59, 61
Altruism 93
'Amount of specification' 58
Ampere 43
Ampere's neologism 42
Amplifying indeterminacy 109
  intelligence 115
Analogue computers 105
Analogue signal 48
Anarchists 7, 8
'And' gate 29, 61, 63, 79, 101, 123, 127
'And' gate with tolerance 61
Andreski 115
Andresky, Professor 164
Anologies 14, 32, 130
Anthropocentrism 38
Anthropomorphic 31, 117, 146
  philosophies 105
Apical 28, 68, 160
  regions 68, 91, 101, 129, 150, 164
  segments 73
Apices 57, 59, 68, 87, 89, 92, 100, 101, 102, 113, 149, 158, 169, 173
Appetite(s) 30, 89, 95, 118, 119, 120
  Balance 89
Ardrey 154, 164
Aristocracy 157
Arousal 89, 98, 118, 119, 147, 170
Artificial intelligence 104
Ashby, Ross 13, 47, 117
'Assemblies of Assemblies' 58, 86
Attention 35, 42, 49, 54, 55, 89, 92, 93, 96, 97, 99, 100, 102, 150, 151, 156
  inputs 75
  point 94, 99
Autonomic 101, 146, 147, 149, 156
Autonomous central processes 118
Axiomatic systems 121

Bacon 106, 113
Balance of probabilities 122
'Barrel of apples' 29, 38
Barton's textbook 47
Behaviour-changing 160, 161
Behaviour patterns 21, 26, 28, 29, 30, 31, 57, 80, 87, 94, 95, 99, 101, 133, 134, 138, 141, 143
Behavioural science 31, 105
Behaviourist 55, 95
Bergson 106
'Big gang' 12
Bigelow 42
Biological recognition 54, 61, 66, 119
Biomass 38, 168
Biomorphic 104, 115, 154, 163
  philosophy 104
  thinking 111
Bionic 154
'Bionics' 43
Biosimulation 104
Biosphere 29, 38, 47, 168
Bourgeois 114
Black box 32, 46, 48, 49, 70, 77, 95
Brain 7, 8, 9, 11, 12, 17, 19, 21, 24,

26, 27, 29, 30, 32, 37, 46, 48, 50, 68, 70, 73, 75, 77, 85, 88, 89, 91, 92, 95, 99, 104, 120, 122, 129, 130, 132, 133, 135, 141, 142, 149, 150, 151, 158, 160, 164, 168, 175
British National Physical Laboratory 131
Bronowski 164
Built-in obsolescence 40
Burt, Professor Sir Cyril 115, 155, 164

Caldwell 42
Capitalist system 159
Catholic church 136
Central decision 50, 57, 89, 153, 158
Centrocephalic 91
Cell-assembly 76
Cerebral cortex 89, 91
Cervantes 22
Change-accepting mechanisms 22
Change-offering mechanisms 21, 30, 33
Change-resisting system 44
Charrette 43, 43n.
Chocolate drop 120, 121, 127
Churchill 115
Class-bias 114
Class boundaries 67
Clockwork universe 106
Cohen, Dr Jack 38
Comfort, Dr Alex 39
Commercial firm 45
Communication 15, 149, 168
Communism 109, 172
Computers 31, 32, 61, 153, 160
Conation 89
Configuration of signal 46
Configurations 37, 155
Confirmation and falsification 117
Consciousness 89
Conservatism 33, 35, 172
 and conservation 133
Conservative 8, 133, 136
Consumerist 9
Contradictory stimuli 91
Control 11
Convergence 44, 50, 57
Convergent 55, 59, 76
Copernicus 129
Cortex 22, 57, 75, 91, 127, 150
Coordinated morphostasis 19
Cross-fertilization of knowledge 32
Cultural heredities 26
Cyberneticist 32, 115
Cybernetics 14, 15, 31, 42, 43, 95, 104, 111
Cybernetics Congress 43, 79
Cytoplasm 23, 75

Darlington 114, 115, 134, 140
Darwin 111, 114
Data Bank 96
Decision 50, 51, 52, 53, 54, 55, 59, 61, 62, 75, 76, 78, 101, 145, 151, 153, 157, 163, 165
 centres 39, 76, 81, 85, 139, 147, 160, 161, 164, 165, 170, 171, 173
 making 32, 45, 48, 155, 156
'Déjà vu' 99
Dendrites 68, 85, 88, 125, 128
Dendritic connections 125
 end 126
 program 126
Descartes 95, 106, 113
Deterioration 40
Determinacy 95
Determinism 94, 106, 111
Determinist 175
Deterministic 114
 computers 61
 thinking 128
Diencephalon 91
Diploid 22
Dirac 107
Discrimination 126
Distal communication 86
 reinforcement 81
Divergence 28, 50, 144
Divergent 59, 76

Eccles 155, 175, 176
Ecology 10, 153
Ecological Balance 134
 niche 26, 29, 30, 36, 40, 96
Economic Boom 110
Economies 108
Eddington 12, 44, 48
Educability 109

'Effectors' 27, 28, 32, 45, 48, 49, 142, 157
Efferent 32, 48, 49, 50, 63, 69, 76, 81, 85, 87, 88, 89, 100, 101, 125, 136, 139, 143, 144
cascade 88
Ego 89, 93, 97, 99, 156
Einstein 129
Elite 10, 158, 168
Embryonic development 21
Encyclopaedists 115
'Enough' gate 68, 70, 82
Entropy 12, 13, 14, 16, 39, 40, 46, 77, 149
Environment 13, 21, 22, 29, 30, 31, 32, 36, 47, 95, 149, 154
Epistemological 12, 44, 104, 110
theory 42
Epistemology 77, 104
Equiponderous 39, 47, 109, 157, 166
Equipotentiality 37, 70, 119
Errors of exclusion 67
of inclusion 67
Ethologists 134
Euler 53
Eureka feeling 7
Evocative 102
Excitability of currencies 110
Excitatory 63, 160
Experimentation 21
Eysenck 38, 115, 164

Falsification 154
Feedback 9, 17, 102, 138, 141, 149
Figure recognition 79, 131
First World War 113
Fisher, R. A. 39
Flow of information 45, 160
Forester, C. S. 141
Free will 94
Fremlin, Professor 165
Freud 108
Freudians 114
Fussiness 125

Galton 115
Ganglion cells 73
Gate(s) 8, 28, 61, 62, 63, 66, 67, 68, 71, 75, 76, 87, 96, 97, 100, 125, 126, 127, 129, 158
Generalization 68, 73, 129
gates 68, 129
Geneticists 35
Genetics 94, 156
Gestalt 46, 78
Gestalters 78, 130
Ginsberg 110
Glial cells 130
Goedel 77
Goedel's theorem 122
Good, I. J. 133
Good, Professor John 117, 164
'Governor' 43
Green, Professor R. T. 164
'Growth' 34, 159

Haploid 21, 22
Hebb 69
Hegel 109, 113
Heisenberg 107, 132, 175
Heracleitas 15
Hierarchic 28, 35, 55, 67, 76, 143
Hierarchical 57, 89, 119, 143
Hierarchy(-ies) 57, 69, 84, 87, 89, 101, 102, 126, 130, 139, 142, 144, 146, 147, 153, 160, 175
High specification 119
Hitler 162
Hobbes 34, 106, 113
Homeostat 43
Homeostasis 16, 17, 35
Homeostatic 13, 15, 20
systems 15
Homo faber 106
Homologous 37, 77, 96, 175
Homologue 17, 44, 147, 156, 175
Hubel, D. H. 73, 119
Human intelligence 39
Hume 113
Huxley, Julian 29, 38, 115
Hyde, Wilfred 164, 165
Hypnot, M. 38

Imagination 99
Improbable arrangement 45
Independent variables 52
Indeterminacy 26, 94
Indeterminism 95, 155, 175
Inferences 96
Information 8, 9, 17, 20, 21, 22, 23,

26, 27, 28, 31, 32, 33, 36, 37, 42, 44, 45, 47, 48, 49, 51, 54, 55, 57, 59, 61, 67, 68, 70, 75, 76, 77, 81, 82, 89, 91, 95, 101, 144, 146, 149, 151, 152, 15?, 157, 158, 160, 165, 171
sources 81
system 24, 44, 48
theory 31, 42, 44, 111, 129
Inhibitive 62
signals 66
Instability of attention 119
Intelligence 9, 10, 11, 20, 22, 24, 26, 29, 37, 38, 46, 109, 139, 167, 173
explosion 133
gap 9
Intelligent 7, 9, 10, 115, 168, 172
Intelligentsia 112
Intellectual 112, 113, 167, 169
Intensity 59
Intention 89
'Intention tremor' 31
Interdisciplinary discipline 43
science 42, 43
Internal attention 97

Jackson, Hughlings 91
Jasper, Sir Herbert 91
Jung 108

Kant 113, 114, 122
Kapp, Professor 117
Karl 128
Keith, Sir Arthur 134
Kepler 129
Knossos 97
Koestler 11
Kropotkin 8, 155

Lashley 119
Lateral communication 84, 86
inhibition 81, 82
Leakey 106
Learning 80, 154
'Learns' 22, 94
Loci 21, 22, 27, 58, 59, 63, 68, 73, 87, 91, 99, 119, 120, 129
Locke 113
Locus 8, 27, 57, 58, 61, 63, 129, 158
Longevity 40
Lorenz 115, 140, 141
Lower sufficiency 66, 129
Low specification 119

Macrocosm 111
Malatesta 8, 155
Malinowsky 134
'Mammal Man', The 37
Management 11
Marx, Beppo 103
Groucho 103
Marx, Karl 109, 113, 155
Marxism, Marxist views 114, 161, 167
Maxwell 20
'Maxwell's demon' 20, 45, 47
McCulloch 42
Mead, Margaret 134
Meaning 58
Mechanomorphic 106, 107, 128
hypotheses 108
philosophies 106
thinking 110, 112, 114
Medewar 115
Memory 97, 99, 118
centre 99, 118
Mesencephalon 91
Mesocosm 111, 175, 176
Metahomeostatic 8, 15
Meta-Morphostatis 33
Metaprogram 125, 126, 127
Metazoa 14, 15, 21, 22, 26
Meter readings 48
Microcosm 111, 176
Microcosmic 47, 175
Microhomologue 17, 45, 47
Model 105
Model making 104
'Models' 32
'Molecule' 20, 45, 47
Money 160, 161, 162
Monohierarchic 70, 141, 142, 143, 147, 152, 153, 156, 162, 167, 170, 171
Monolinear 102, 132, 164
chains 44
Montaigne 106
Morphoretention 13
Morphoretentor 14
Morphostatis 13, 33

Morphostat(s) 14, 17, 20, 32, 33, 46, 115, 130, 140, 141, 152, 157, 159, 175
Morphostatic 14, 17, 21, 22, 30, 32, 34, 37, 118, 142, 155, 171, 173
Morris 164
Mother Nature 173
Motoneurons 149
Motorium 23, 27, 50, 53, 69, 70, 75, 76, 85, 86, 87, 89, 94, 127, 137, 144, 150, 151, 153, 161, 164, 165, 168
Multilinear 102
  input 76
  systems 44
Multiplexing 69, 129
Muscle spindles 49
Mutants 35

Nader 153
Natural Goodness of Man 9
Negentropy 13, 14, 29, 47
Neologism 14, 57
Neumann, von 42
Neuron 8, 128, 129, 132
Neurophysiology 42, 69
New Guinea 134
Newton 113
Non-Morphostatic 30

Object comparate 53, 54, 55, 58, 59, 61, 66, 71
Odds balancing 39
'One-thing-at-a-time' strategy 89
Ontogenetic 24, 118
  intelligence 29, 30
Operation research 31
Org(s) 14, 15, 17, 18, 19, 28, 29, 31, 32, 33, 34, 36, 37, 39, 40, 44, 45, 46, 47, 48, 49, 51, 52, 53, 61, 68, 69, 75, 76, 80, 89, 95, 101, 110, 121, 125, 130, 135, 136, 140, 141, 144, 147, 150, 159, 161, 164, 165, 171
Organization 7, 9, 11, 31, 32, 34, 35, 36, 37, 74, 81, 101, 102, 140, 141, 142, 143, 144, 146, 147, 149, 150, 152, 154, 155, 156, 157, 160, 168, 170
'Or' Gate 63, 68, 71, 112, 118, 123
Orthodox thought shackles 113
Out-of-date gods and kings 113

Pascal's Law 67
Parks, Dr 79, 131
Parameters 38, 46, 52, 53
Pattern recognition 62, 104, 123, 131, 133
Pavlov 55
Penfield 89, 91, 131, 157
Perception 51, 52, 61, 94, 96, 99, 100, 119, 150
Percepts 52, 55, 58, 59, 61, 63, 66, 68, 69, 96, 97
Perceptual elements 57, 58, 59, 62, 63, 69, 70, 73, 74, 79, 86, 119, 120, 127, 131
Permissible deviation 52
Philosophy of Science Journal 128
Phylogenetic (-ally) 24, 29, 30, 31
  intelligent 30
Planck 107
Planning 101
Pleasure-pain 26, 30, 85, 159
Plethora 42, 160
Pitts 42
Point intensities 50
Polyak 119
Polycentric system 150
Polyhierarchies 89
Polyhierarchic 57, 61, 63, 66, 67, 68, 70, 73, 74, 77, 80, 81, 128, 142, 143, 144, 146, 149, 151, 152, 153, 155, 156, 160, 164, 170, 171, 172
  Apices 91
  connectional network 123
  divergent flow 115
  hypothesis 119
  information 89, 123
  network 57, 59, 66, 69, 70, 86, 142, 150, 158, 171
  structure 59, 70, 147, 161
  systems 80, 81, 86, 135, 161, 170
Popper 110, 121, 122, 128
Positive feedback 44
Post-lateral gyri 73
'Poverty of Historicism' 110
Power 17, 31, 157
Predators 40
Prediction 131

Predictive system 77
Predictors 31
Presentation 73
Pressure 109
'Probability' 12
Program boxes 125
Proprioceptive 75, 149, 153
information 91
receptors 49
Protozoa 15, 21
Proudhon 8, 155
Psychology 39, 108
Psychometrics 158, 162
Psychometrists 109
Psycho-physical dualism 104
Ptolomaic astronomic model 129
Pure Science 163
Pure Scientist 164

Quixotic sub-goals 93

Randomness 80, 95, 119
Random numbers 125, 126
Ratiocination 95, 96
'Reaction' 35
Receptor(s) 17, 26, 27, 28, 29, 34, 45, 46, 48, 49, 51, 52, 55, 57, 59, 63, 70, 75, 76, 82, 84, 85, 95, 119, 125, 136, 142, 157
Recessive genes 94
'Recognized' 58
Recognizable 112
Recognition 52, 54, 55, 57, 58, 61, 66, 67, 68, 73, 87, 129, 131
Recombination 68
Register 59, 73
Reith lectures 139
Relevant information 75
Repertoire 21, 26, 30, 76, 142, 143, 157
Reticular formation 89
Retina 17, 49, 57, 66, 86, 87, 120
Roberts 91
Role allocation 9, 158
Rotation 61
Rousseau 115, 158
Russell, Bertrand 42

Sapience 11, 44, 46
Satisfaction 118
Senility 14, 39, 40
Scale 59
Schon, Professor 34, 139
Science, epistemological nature of, 12
Scientist 11, 44, 113
Self-reinforcing circuits 119
Semantic filter 68
pattern 102
Sensorium 23, 27, 63, 50, 51, 52, 53, 55, 57, 58, 59, 66, 70, 75, 76, 82, 86, 87, 89, 94, 113, 123, 125, 126, 137, 142, 144, 150, 152, 153, 164, 165
Serebriakoff's Law 41
Servo mechanisms 31
Set 14, 89
Shannon, 42, 115
Shaw 158
Signal(s) 9, 17, 20, 21, 27, 31, 45, 52, 53, 57, 58, 63, 73, 77, 78, 81, 87, 102, 144, 153, 157, 160
and information 45
Significance 87
Skinner 55, 95
Skinnerians 95
Slump 110
Social reward 159, 172
Sociological intelligence 26
Sociology 108, 109
Spearman 115
Specification 53, 66, 67, 129
Spenser 113, 114
Spenserian 115
Spontaneous firing 119
Stability 40, 47, 160
-seeking 34, 45, 133
Statistical laws 39
Stochastic 132
computers 133
Subject comparate 53, 54, 55, 59, 61, 66
Subject and object comparates 61
'Success' 32, 125
signal 86
Success measurement 30
Sufficiency 54, 62, 63, 66, 67, 68, 75, 82, 89, 125, 126, 127
gate 61, 63, 79, 123, 127, 130
Sumer 106

Summation 44, 55
Super-org 135, 168, 171
Strategic 95
Symbiotic 134, 160, 173
Synapses 68
Synaptic box 125
Synergistic effects 74

Tactical 95
Tarzan 37
Teleological 45
Teleologically 28, 32
Temperature 20, 109
Tendons 49
Terman 115
Territorial imperative 164
Theory of information 42
Thermodynamics 109
    second law of 12, 13, 20, 46, 47
Theseus 97
Thick cybernetics 108
Third order intelligence 31, 36
'Threshold' gates 62
Tinbergen 115
Tolerance 45, 46, 52, 53, 54, 61, 62, 63, 66, 67, 77, 119, 129
Transducer 21
Trends 116
Trigger 20, 29, 32
'Trigger Action' 17, 20, 50, 100
Tungsten micro-electrodes 73
Turing 42

Ubiquitous signal 125, 130
Uncertainty-amplifying 175
Undeterministic 45
Undeveloped country 104
Unfalsifiable propositions 117
Utopia 113

'Vague, verbal, unpredictive models' 110
Variables 45
Vector 54
Vectorial 53
Vertebrae 29
Visual cortex 55
Vocalization 131
Volatile minds 94
Volition 82, 89
Volitional 85, 94, 99, 100, 101
    centre 92
Von Foerster, Heinz, 79, 115
Volition 89
Volume 109
'Voting' gates 62

Walter, Gray, 132
Wells, H. G. 158
Whewell 111
Whim 95, 155, 175
White swan controversy 128
Whole situation requiring action 102
Wiener, Norbert 12, 13, 14, 31, 42, 43, 45, 55, 115
Wiesel, T. N. 73, 119
Wide tolerance 66
    recognition 131
World Brain 110, 168, 173
    Motorium 172
    Org 169, 170, 172
    society 110

Young, J. Z. 115